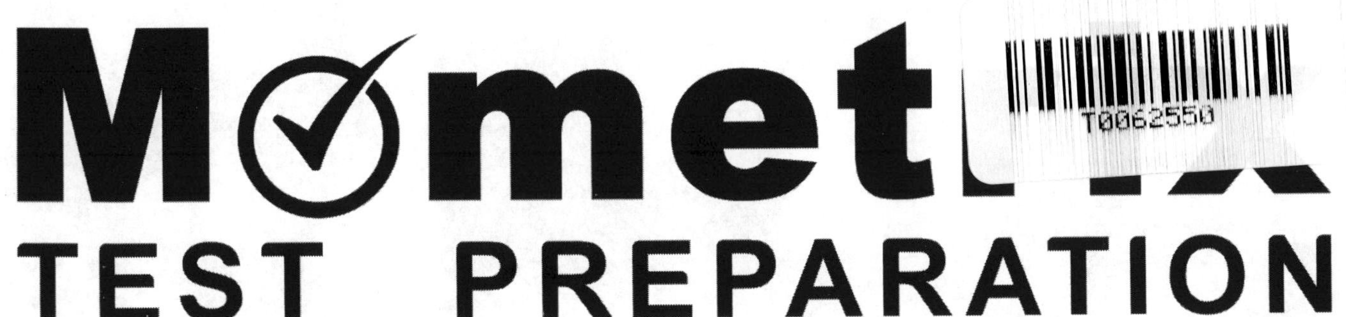

Medical Lab Assistant

Exam Secrets Study Guide

DEAR FUTURE EXAM SUCCESS STORY

First of all, **THANK YOU** for purchasing Mometrix study materials!

Second, congratulations! You are one of the few determined test-takers who are committed to doing whatever it takes to excel on your exam. **You have come to the right place.** We developed these study materials with one goal in mind: to deliver you the information you need in a format that's concise and easy to use.

In addition to optimizing your guide for the content of the test, we've outlined our recommended steps for breaking down the preparation process into small, attainable goals so you can make sure you stay on track.

We've also analyzed the entire test-taking process, identifying the most common pitfalls and showing how you can overcome them and be ready for any curveball the test throws you.

Standardized testing is one of the biggest obstacles on your road to success, which only increases the importance of doing well in the high-pressure, high-stakes environment of test day. Your results on this test could have a significant impact on your future, and this guide provides the information and practical advice to help you achieve your full potential on test day.

Your success is our success

We would love to hear from you! If you would like to share the story of your exam success or if you have any questions or comments in regard to our products, please contact us at **800-673-8175** or **support@mometrix.com**.

Thanks again for your business and we wish you continued success!

Sincerely,
The Mometrix Test Preparation Team

Need more help? Check out our flashcards at:
http://MometrixFlashcards.com/MedicalLabAssistant

Written and edited by the Mometrix Exam Secrets Test Prep Team
Printed in the United States of America

Table of Contents

Introduction

Thank you for purchasing this resource! You have made the choice to prepare yourself for a test that could have a huge impact on your future, and this guide is designed to help you be fully ready for test day. Obviously, it's important to have a solid understanding of the test material, but you also need to be prepared for the unique environment and stressors of the test, so that you can perform to the best of your abilities.

For this purpose, the first section that appears in this guide is the **Secret Keys**. We've devoted countless hours to meticulously researching what works and what doesn't, and we've boiled down our findings to the five most impactful steps you can take to improve your performance on the test. We start at the beginning with study planning and move through the preparation process, all the way to the testing strategies that will help you get the most out of what you know when you're finally sitting in front of the test.

We recommend that you start preparing for your test as far in advance as possible. However, if you've bought this guide as a last-minute study resource and only have a few days before your test, we recommend that you skip over the first two Secret Keys since they address a long-term study plan.

If you struggle with **test anxiety**, we strongly encourage you to check out our recommendations for how you can overcome it. Test anxiety is a formidable foe, but it can be beaten, and we want to make sure you have the tools you need to defeat it.

Secret Key #1 – Plan Big, Study Small

There's a lot riding on your performance. If you want to ace this test, you're going to need to keep your skills sharp and the material fresh in your mind. You need a plan that lets you review everything you need to know while still fitting in your schedule. We'll break this strategy down into three categories.

Information Organization

Start with the information you already have: the official test outline. From this, you can make a complete list of all the concepts you need to cover before the test. Organize these concepts into groups that can be studied together, and create a list of any related vocabulary you need to learn so you can brush up on any difficult terms. You'll want to keep this vocabulary list handy once you actually start studying since you may need to add to it along the way.

Time Management

Once you have your set of study concepts, decide how to spread them out over the time you have left before the test. Break your study plan into small, clear goals so you have a manageable task for each day and know exactly what you're doing. Then just focus on one small step at a time. When you manage your time this way, you don't need to spend hours at a time studying. Studying a small block of content for a short period each day helps you retain information better and avoid stressing over how much you have left to do. You can relax knowing that you have a plan to cover everything in time. In order for this strategy to be effective though, you have to start studying early and stick to your schedule. Avoid the exhaustion and futility that comes from last-minute cramming!

Study Environment

The environment you study in has a big impact on your learning. Studying in a coffee shop, while probably more enjoyable, is not likely to be as fruitful as studying in a quiet room. It's important to keep distractions to a minimum. You're only planning to study for a short block of time, so make the most of it. Don't pause to check your phone or get up to find a snack. It's also important to **avoid multitasking**. Research has consistently shown that multitasking will make your studying dramatically less effective. Your study area should also be comfortable and well-lit so you don't have the distraction of straining your eyes or sitting on an uncomfortable chair.

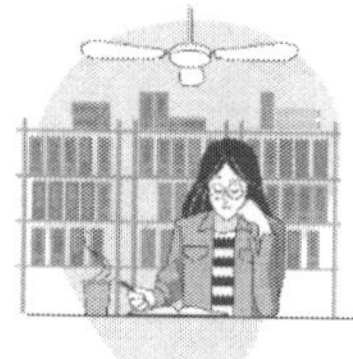

The time of day you study is also important. You want to be rested and alert. Don't wait until just before bedtime. Study when you'll be most likely to comprehend and remember. Even better, if you know what time of day your test will be, set that time aside for study. That way your brain will be used to working on that subject at that specific time and you'll have a better chance of recalling information.

Finally, it can be helpful to team up with others who are studying for the same test. Your actual studying should be done in as isolated an environment as possible, but the work of organizing the information and setting up the study plan can be divided up. In between study sessions, you can discuss with your teammates the concepts that you're all studying and quiz each other on the details. Just be sure that your teammates are as serious about the test as you are. If you find that your study time is being replaced with social time, you might need to find a new team.

Secret Key #2 – Make Your Studying Count

You're devoting a lot of time and effort to preparing for this test, so you want to be absolutely certain it will pay off. This means doing more than just reading the content and hoping you can remember it on test day. It's important to make every minute of study count. There are two main areas you can focus on to make your studying count.

Retention

It doesn't matter how much time you study if you can't remember the material. You need to make sure you are retaining the concepts. To check your retention of the information you're learning, try recalling it at later times with minimal prompting. Try carrying around flashcards and glance at one or two from time to time or ask a friend who's also studying for the test to quiz you.

To enhance your retention, look for ways to put the information into practice so that you can apply it rather than simply recalling it. If you're using the information in practical ways, it will be much easier to remember. Similarly, it helps to solidify a concept in your mind if you're not only reading it to yourself but also explaining it to someone else. Ask a friend to let you teach them about a concept you're a little shaky on (or speak aloud to an imaginary audience if necessary). As you try to summarize, define, give examples, and answer your friend's questions, you'll understand the concepts better and they will stay with you longer. Finally, step back for a big picture view and ask yourself how each piece of information fits with the whole subject. When you link the different concepts together and see them working together as a whole, it's easier to remember the individual components.

Finally, practice showing your work on any multi-step problems, even if you're just studying. Writing out each step you take to solve a problem will help solidify the process in your mind, and you'll be more likely to remember it during the test.

Modality

Modality simply refers to the means or method by which you study. Choosing a study modality that fits your own individual learning style is crucial. No two people learn best in exactly the same way, so it's important to know your strengths and use them to your advantage.

For example, if you learn best by visualization, focus on visualizing a concept in your mind and draw an image or a diagram. Try color-coding your notes, illustrating them, or creating symbols that will trigger your mind to recall a learned concept. If you learn best by hearing or discussing information, find a study partner who learns the same way or read aloud to yourself. Think about how to put the information in your own words. Imagine that you are giving a lecture on the topic and record yourself so you can listen to it later.

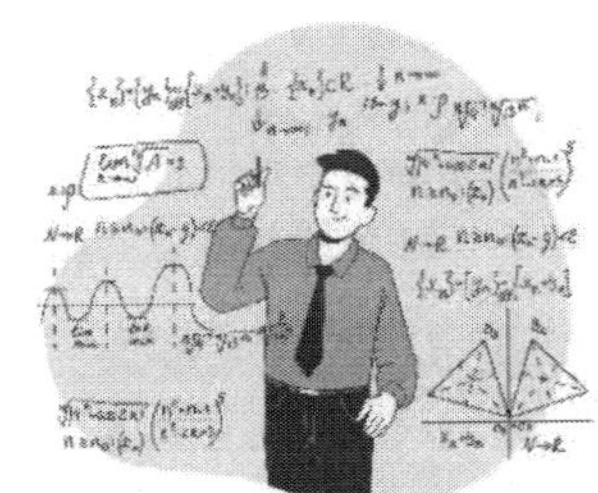

For any learning style, flashcards can be helpful. Organize the information so you can take advantage of spare moments to review. Underline key words or phrases. Use different colors for different categories. Mnemonic devices (such as creating a short list in which every item starts with the same letter) can also help with retention. Find what works best for you and use it to store the information in your mind most effectively and easily.

Secret Key #3 – Practice the Right Way

Your success on test day depends not only on how many hours you put into preparing, but also on whether you prepared the right way. It's good to check along the way to see if your studying is paying off. One of the most effective ways to do this is by taking practice tests to evaluate your progress. Practice tests are useful because they show exactly where you need to improve. Every time you take a practice test, pay special attention to these three groups of questions:

- The questions you got wrong
- The questions you had to guess on, even if you guessed right
- The questions you found difficult or slow to work through

This will show you exactly what your weak areas are, and where you need to devote more study time. Ask yourself why each of these questions gave you trouble. Was it because you didn't understand the material? Was it because you didn't remember the vocabulary? Do you need more repetitions on this type of question to build speed and confidence? Dig into those questions and figure out how you can strengthen your weak areas as you go back to review the material.

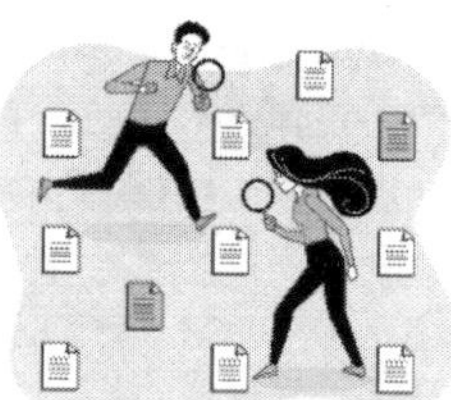

Additionally, many practice tests have a section explaining the answer choices. It can be tempting to read the explanation and think that you now have a good understanding of the concept. However, an explanation likely only covers part of the question's broader context. Even if the explanation makes perfect sense, **go back and investigate** every concept related to the question until you're positive you have a thorough understanding.

As you go along, keep in mind that the practice test is just that: practice. Memorizing these questions and answers will not be very helpful on the actual test because it is unlikely to have any of the same exact questions. If you only know the right answers to the sample questions, you won't be prepared for the real thing. **Study the concepts** until you understand them fully, and then you'll be able to answer any question that shows up on the test.

It's important to wait on the practice tests until you're ready. If you take a test on your first day of study, you may be overwhelmed by the amount of material covered and how much you need to learn. Work up to it gradually.

On test day, you'll need to be prepared for answering questions, managing your time, and using the test-taking strategies you've learned. It's a lot to balance, like a mental marathon that will have a big impact on your future. Like training for a marathon, you'll need to start slowly and work your way up. When test day arrives, you'll be ready.

Start with the strategies you've read in the first two Secret Keys—plan your course and study in the way that works best for you. If you have time, consider using multiple study resources to get different approaches to the same concepts. It can be helpful to see difficult concepts from more than one angle. Then find a good source for practice tests. Many times, the test website will suggest potential study resources or provide sample tests.

Practice Test Strategy

If you're able to find at least three practice tests, we recommend this strategy:

Untimed and Open-Book Practice

Take the first test with no time constraints and with your notes and study guide handy. Take your time and focus on applying the strategies you've learned.

Timed and Open-Book Practice

Take the second practice test open-book as well, but set a timer and practice pacing yourself to finish in time.

Timed and Closed-Book Practice

Take any other practice tests as if it were test day. Set a timer and put away your study materials. Sit at a table or desk in a quiet room, imagine yourself at the testing center, and answer questions as quickly and accurately as possible.

Keep repeating timed and closed-book tests on a regular basis until you run out of practice tests or it's time for the actual test. Your mind will be ready for the schedule and stress of test day, and you'll be able to focus on recalling the material you've learned.

Secret Key #4 – Pace Yourself

Once you're fully prepared for the material on the test, your biggest challenge on test day will be managing your time. Just knowing that the clock is ticking can make you panic even if you have plenty of time left. Work on pacing yourself so you can build confidence against the time constraints of the exam. Pacing is a difficult skill to master, especially in a high-pressure environment, so **practice is vital**.

Set time expectations for your pace based on how much time is available. For example, if a section has 60 questions and the time limit is 30 minutes, you know you have to average 30 seconds or less per question in order to answer them all. Although 30 seconds is the hard limit, set 25 seconds per question as your goal, so you reserve extra time to spend on harder questions. When you budget extra time for the harder questions, you no longer have any reason to stress when those questions take longer to answer.

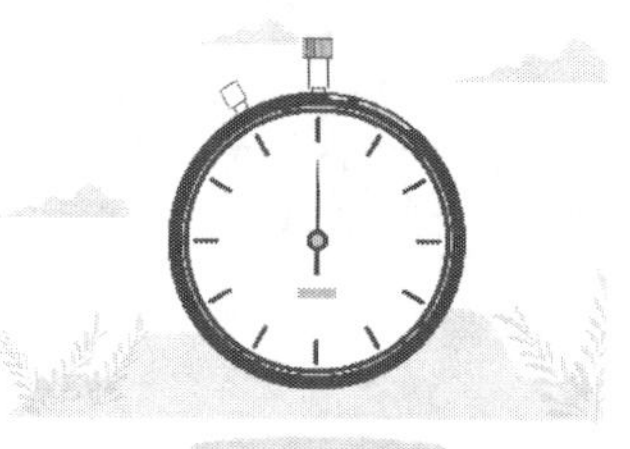

Don't let this time expectation distract you from working through the test at a calm, steady pace, but keep it in mind so you don't spend too much time on any one question. Recognize that taking extra time on one question you don't understand may keep you from answering two that you do understand later in the test. If your time limit for a question is up and you're still not sure of the answer, mark it and move on, and come back to it later if the time and the test format allow. If the testing format doesn't allow you to return to earlier questions, just make an educated guess; then put it out of your mind and move on.

On the easier questions, be careful not to rush. It may seem wise to hurry through them so you have more time for the challenging ones, but it's not worth missing one if you know the concept and just didn't take the time to read the question fully. Work efficiently but make sure you understand the question and have looked at all of the answer choices, since more than one may seem right at first.

Even if you're paying attention to the time, you may find yourself a little behind at some point. You should speed up to get back on track, but do so wisely. Don't panic; just take a few seconds less on each question until you're caught up. Don't guess without thinking, but do look through the answer choices and eliminate any you know are wrong. If you can get down to two choices, it is often worthwhile to guess from those. Once you've chosen an answer, move on and don't dwell on any that you skipped or had to hurry through. If a question was taking too long, chances are it was one of the harder ones, so you weren't as likely to get it right anyway.

On the other hand, if you find yourself getting ahead of schedule, it may be beneficial to slow down a little. The more quickly you work, the more likely you are to make a careless mistake that will affect your score. You've budgeted time for each question, so don't be afraid to spend that time. Practice an efficient but careful pace to get the most out of the time you have.

Secret Key #5 – Have a Plan for Guessing

When you're taking the test, you may find yourself stuck on a question. Some of the answer choices seem better than others, but you don't see the one answer choice that is obviously correct. What do you do?

The scenario described above is very common, yet most test takers have not effectively prepared for it. Developing and practicing a plan for guessing may be one of the single most effective uses of your time as you get ready for the exam.

In developing your plan for guessing, there are three questions to address:

- When should you start the guessing process?
- How should you narrow down the choices?
- Which answer should you choose?

When to Start the Guessing Process

Unless your plan for guessing is to select C every time (which, despite its merits, is not what we recommend), you need to leave yourself enough time to apply your answer elimination strategies. Since you have a limited amount of time for each question, that means that if you're going to give yourself the best shot at guessing correctly, you have to decide quickly whether or not you will guess.

Of course, the best-case scenario is that you don't have to guess at all, so first, see if you can answer the question based on your knowledge of the subject and basic reasoning skills. Focus on the key words in the question and try to jog your memory of related topics. Give yourself a chance to bring the knowledge to mind, but once you realize that you don't have (or you can't access) the knowledge you need to answer the question, it's time to start the guessing process.

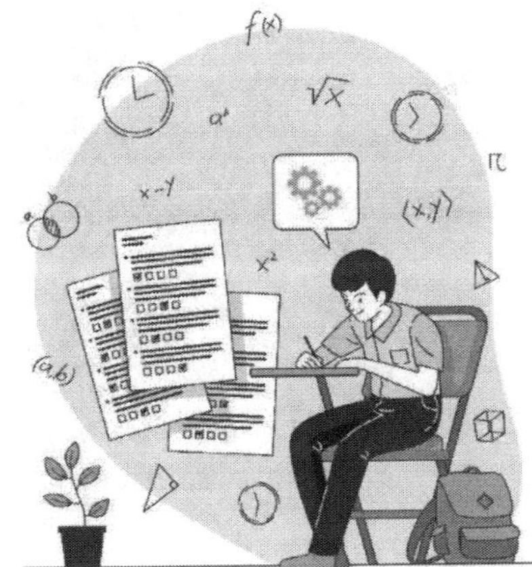

It's almost always better to start the guessing process too early than too late. It only takes a few seconds to remember something and answer the question from knowledge. Carefully eliminating wrong answer choices takes longer. Plus, going through the process of eliminating answer choices can actually help jog your memory.

Summary: Start the guessing process as soon as you decide that you can't answer the question based on your knowledge.

How to Narrow Down the Choices

The next chapter in this book (**Test-Taking Strategies**) includes a wide range of strategies for how to approach questions and how to look for answer choices to eliminate. You will definitely want to read those carefully, practice them, and figure out which ones work best for you. Here though, we're going to address a mindset rather than a particular strategy.

Your odds of guessing an answer correctly depend on how many options you are choosing from.

Number of options left	5	4	3	2	1
Odds of guessing correctly	20%	25%	33%	50%	100%

You can see from this chart just how valuable it is to be able to eliminate incorrect answers and make an educated guess, but there are two things that many test takers do that cause them to miss out on the benefits of guessing:

- Accidentally eliminating the correct answer
- Selecting an answer based on an impression

We'll look at the first one here, and the second one in the next section.

To avoid accidentally eliminating the correct answer, we recommend a thought exercise called **the $5 challenge**. In this challenge, you only eliminate an answer choice from contention if you are willing to bet $5 on it being wrong. Why $5? Five dollars is a small but not insignificant amount of money. It's an amount you could afford to lose but wouldn't want to throw away. And while losing $5 once might not hurt too much, doing it twenty times will set you back $100. In the same way, each small decision you make—eliminating a choice here, guessing on a question there—won't by itself impact your score very much, but when you put them all together, they can make a big difference. By holding each answer choice elimination decision to a higher standard, you can reduce the risk of accidentally eliminating the correct answer.

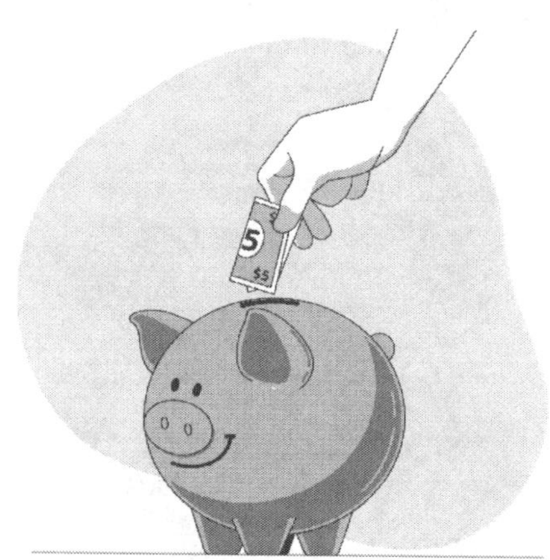

The $5 challenge can also be applied in a positive sense: If you are willing to bet $5 that an answer choice *is* correct, go ahead and mark it as correct.

Summary: Only eliminate an answer choice if you are willing to bet $5 that it is wrong.

Which Answer to Choose

You're taking the test. You've run into a hard question and decided you'll have to guess. You've eliminated all the answer choices you're willing to bet $5 on. Now you have to pick an answer. Why do we even need to talk about this? Why can't you just pick whichever one you feel like when the time comes?

The answer to these questions is that if you don't come into the test with a plan, you'll rely on your impression to select an answer choice, and if you do that, you risk falling into a trap. The test writers know that everyone who takes their test will be guessing on some of the questions, so they intentionally write wrong answer choices to seem plausible. You still have to pick an answer though, and if the wrong answer choices are designed to look right, how can you ever be sure that you're not falling for their trap? The best solution we've found to this dilemma is to take the decision out of your hands entirely. Here is the process we recommend:

Once you've eliminated any choices that you are confident (willing to bet $5) are wrong, select the first remaining choice as your answer.

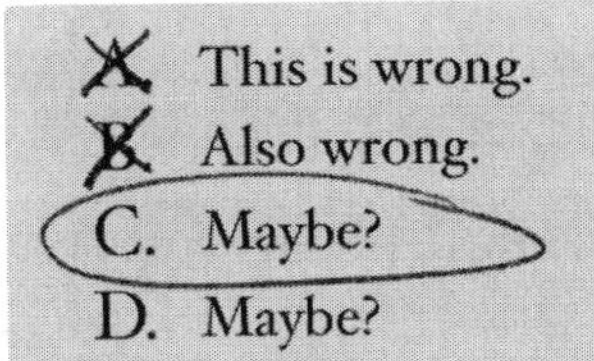

Whether you choose to select the first remaining choice, the second, or the last, the important thing is that you use some preselected standard. Using this approach guarantees that you will not be enticed into selecting an answer choice that looks right, because you are not basing your decision on how the answer choices look.

This is not meant to make you question your knowledge. Instead, it is to help you recognize the difference between your knowledge and your impressions. There's a huge difference between thinking an answer is right because of what you know, and thinking an answer is right because it looks or sounds like it should be right.

Summary: To ensure that your selection is appropriately random, make a predetermined selection from among all answer choices you have not eliminated.

Test-Taking Strategies

This section contains a list of test-taking strategies that you may find helpful as you work through the test. By taking what you know and applying logical thought, you can maximize your chances of answering any question correctly!

It is very important to realize that every question is different and every person is different: no single strategy will work on every question, and no single strategy will work for every person. That's why we've included all of them here, so you can try them out and determine which ones work best for different types of questions and which ones work best for you.

Question Strategies

☑ Read Carefully

Read the question and the answer choices carefully. Don't miss the question because you misread the terms. You have plenty of time to read each question thoroughly and make sure you understand what is being asked. Yet a happy medium must be attained, so don't waste too much time. You must read carefully and efficiently.

☑ Contextual Clues

Look for contextual clues. If the question includes a word you are not familiar with, look at the immediate context for some indication of what the word might mean. Contextual clues can often give you all the information you need to decipher the meaning of an unfamiliar word. Even if you can't determine the meaning, you may be able to narrow down the possibilities enough to make a solid guess at the answer to the question.

☑ Prefixes

If you're having trouble with a word in the question or answer choices, try dissecting it. Take advantage of every clue that the word might include. Prefixes can be a huge help. Usually, they allow you to determine a basic meaning. *Pre-* means before, *post-* means after, *pro-* is positive, *de-* is negative. From prefixes, you can get an idea of the general meaning of the word and try to put it into context.

☑ Hedge Words

Watch out for critical hedge words, such as *likely, may, can, sometimes, often, almost, mostly, usually, generally, rarely,* and *sometimes.* Question writers insert these hedge phrases to cover every possibility. Often an answer choice will be wrong simply because it leaves no room for exception. Be on guard for answer choices that have definitive words such as *exactly* and *always.*

☑ Switchback Words

Stay alert for *switchbacks.* These are the words and phrases frequently used to alert you to shifts in thought. The most common switchback words are *but, although,* and *however.* Others include *nevertheless, on the other hand, even though, while, in spite of, despite,* and *regardless of.* Switchback words are important to catch because they can change the direction of the question or an answer choice.

☑ Face Value

When in doubt, use common sense. Accept the situation in the problem at face value. Don't read too much into it. These problems will not require you to make wild assumptions. If you have to go beyond creativity and warp time or space in order to have an answer choice fit the question, then you should move on and consider the other answer choices. These are normal problems rooted in reality. The applicable relationship or explanation may not be readily apparent, but it is there for you to figure out. Use your common sense to interpret anything that isn't clear.

Answer Choice Strategies

ANSWER SELECTION

The most thorough way to pick an answer choice is to identify and eliminate wrong answers until only one is left, then confirm it is the correct answer. Sometimes an answer choice may immediately seem right, but be careful. The test writers will usually put more than one reasonable answer choice on each question, so take a second to read all of them and make sure that the other choices are not equally obvious. As long as you have time left, it is better to read every answer choice than to pick the first one that looks right without checking the others.

ANSWER CHOICE FAMILIES

An answer choice family consists of two (in rare cases, three) answer choices that are very similar in construction and cannot all be true at the same time. If you see two answer choices that are direct opposites or parallels, one of them is usually the correct answer. For instance, if one answer choice says that quantity *x* increases and another either says that quantity *x* decreases (opposite) or says that quantity *y* increases (parallel), then those answer choices would fall into the same family. An answer choice that doesn't match the construction of the answer choice family is more likely to be incorrect. Most questions will not have answer choice families, but when they do appear, you should be prepared to recognize them.

ELIMINATE ANSWERS

Eliminate answer choices as soon as you realize they are wrong, but make sure you consider all possibilities. If you are eliminating answer choices and realize that the last one you are left with is also wrong, don't panic. Start over and consider each choice again. There may be something you missed the first time that you will realize on the second pass.

AVOID FACT TRAPS

Don't be distracted by an answer choice that is factually true but doesn't answer the question. You are looking for the choice that answers the question. Stay focused on what the question is asking for so you don't accidentally pick an answer that is true but incorrect. Always go back to the question and make sure the answer choice you've selected actually answers the question and is not merely a true statement.

EXTREME STATEMENTS

In general, you should avoid answers that put forth extreme actions as standard practice or proclaim controversial ideas as established fact. An answer choice that states the "process should be used in certain situations, if..." is much more likely to be correct than one that states the "process should be discontinued completely." The first is a calm rational statement and doesn't even make a definitive, uncompromising stance, using a hedge word *if* to provide wiggle room, whereas the second choice is far more extreme.

BENCHMARK

As you read through the answer choices and you come across one that seems to answer the question well, mentally select that answer choice. This is not your final answer, but it's the one that will help you evaluate the other answer choices. The one that you selected is your benchmark or standard for judging each of the other answer choices. Every other answer choice must be compared to your benchmark. That choice is correct until proven otherwise by another answer choice beating it. If you find a better answer, then that one becomes your new benchmark. Once you've decided that no other choice answers the question as well as your benchmark, you have your final answer.

⊘ PREDICT THE ANSWER

Before you even start looking at the answer choices, it is often best to try to predict the answer. When you come up with the answer on your own, it is easier to avoid distractions and traps because you will know exactly what to look for. The right answer choice is unlikely to be word-for-word what you came up with, but it should be a close match. Even if you are confident that you have the right answer, you should still take the time to read each option before moving on.

General Strategies

⊘ TOUGH QUESTIONS

If you are stumped on a problem or it appears too hard or too difficult, don't waste time. Move on! Remember though, if you can quickly check for obviously incorrect answer choices, your chances of guessing correctly are greatly improved. Before you completely give up, at least try to knock out a couple of possible answers. Eliminate what you can and then guess at the remaining answer choices before moving on.

⊘ CHECK YOUR WORK

Since you will probably not know every term listed and the answer to every question, it is important that you get credit for the ones that you do know. Don't miss any questions through careless mistakes. If at all possible, try to take a second to look back over your answer selection and make sure you've selected the correct answer choice and haven't made a costly careless mistake (such as marking an answer choice that you didn't mean to mark). This quick double check should more than pay for itself in caught mistakes for the time it costs.

⊘ PACE YOURSELF

It's easy to be overwhelmed when you're looking at a page full of questions; your mind is confused and full of random thoughts, and the clock is ticking down faster than you would like. Calm down and maintain the pace that you have set for yourself. Especially as you get down to the last few minutes of the test, don't let the small numbers on the clock make you panic. As long as you are on track by monitoring your pace, you are guaranteed to have time for each question.

⊘ DON'T RUSH

It is very easy to make errors when you are in a hurry. Maintaining a fast pace in answering questions is pointless if it makes you miss questions that you would have gotten right otherwise. Test writers like to include distracting information and wrong answers that seem right. Taking a little extra time to avoid careless mistakes can make all the difference in your test score. Find a pace that allows you to be confident in the answers that you select.

⊘ KEEP MOVING

Panicking will not help you pass the test, so do your best to stay calm and keep moving. Taking deep breaths and going through the answer elimination steps you practiced can help to break through a stress barrier and keep your pace.

Final Notes

The combination of a solid foundation of content knowledge and the confidence that comes from practicing your plan for applying that knowledge is the key to maximizing your performance on test day. As your foundation of content knowledge is built up and strengthened, you'll find that the strategies included in this chapter become more and more effective in helping you quickly sift through the distractions and traps of the test to isolate the correct answer.

Now that you're preparing to move forward into the test content chapters of this book, be sure to keep your goal in mind. As you read, think about how you will be able to apply this information on the test. If you've already seen sample questions for the test and you have an idea of the question format and style, try to come up with questions of your own that you can answer based on what you're reading. This will give you valuable practice applying your knowledge in the same ways you can expect to on test day.

Good luck and good studying!

Basic and Relevant Anatomy and Physiology

Skeletal System

Functions

There are about 206 bones in the human body, they function to protect and preserve the shape of soft tissues. The skeleton provides a framework for the muscles, it controls and directs internal pressure and provides stability anchoring points for other soft tissues. There are a wide variety of bones/bony tissues adapted for specific functions to aid locomotion and support; bones are moved by the skeletal muscles. In addition, the skeletal system stores and produces blood cells in the bone marrow.

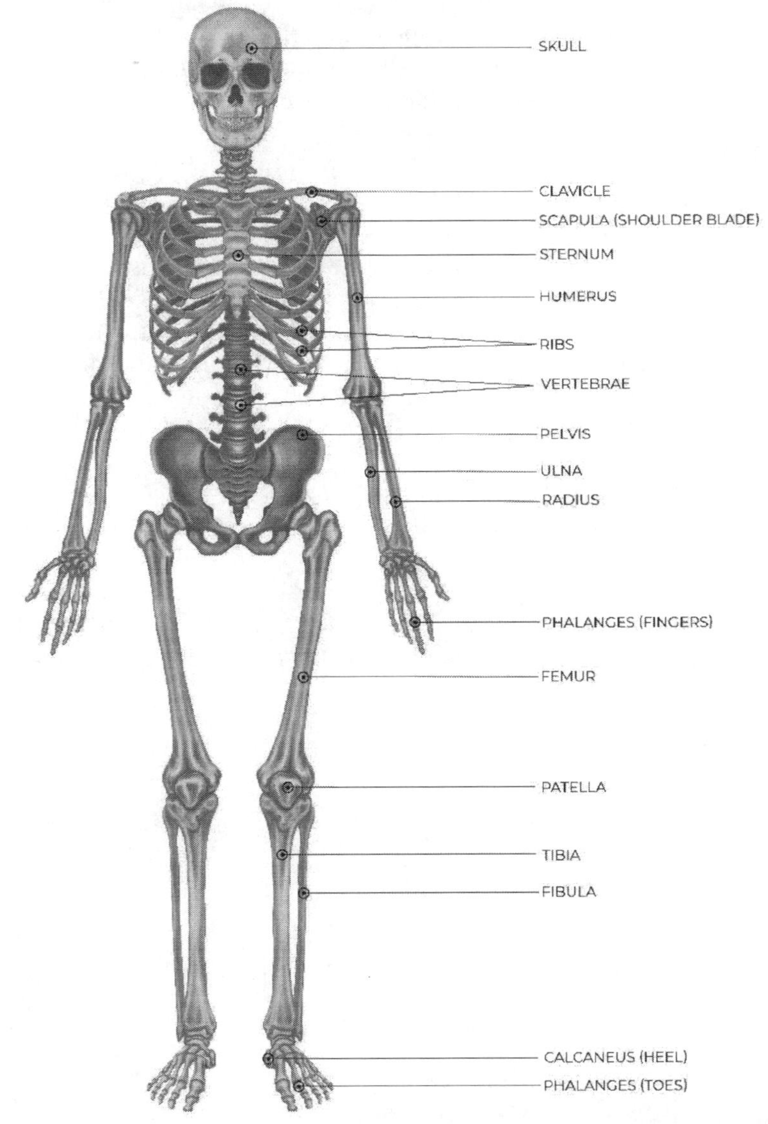

Review Video: Skeletal System
Visit mometrix.com/academy and enter code: 256447

Structures

There are two types of bone tissue: compact and spongy. The names imply that the two types of differ in density, or how tightly the tissue is packed together. There are three types of cells that contribute to bone homeostasis. Osteoblasts are bone-forming cell, osteoclasts resorb or break down bone, and osteocytes are mature bone cells. Equilibrium between osteoblasts and osteoclasts maintains bone tissue.

Bone

Compact

Compact bone is characterized by its structural components: harversian systems or closely packed osteons. Each osteon has a haversian (osteonic) central canal, which is surrounded by a matrix of lamella in concentric ring. The osteocytes (bone cells) are sandwiched between matrix rings in spaces called lacunae. Radiating out from the lacunae are small channels, called canaliculi, which connect the lacunae to the harversian canal, forming passageways through the hard matrix for transport. The harversian systems in compact bone form the appearance of a solid mass because they are so tightly packed. The harversian canals contain blood vessels running parallel to the bone's long axis. Interconnections between these blood vessels and perforating canals link vessels to those on the bone's outer surface.

Spongy

Compared to compact bone, spongy (cancellous) bone is lighter, airier, and less dense. Cancellous bone consists of trabeculae, which are plates and bars of bone, located adjacent to small, irregular red bone marrow-containing cavities. To receive their blood supply, the canaliculi connect with the cavities adjacent to them, rather than the central harversian canal. Although easily mistaken as a having a haphazard appearance, the trabeculae are actually arranged in a particular organization (like braces on a building) that maximizes the bone's strength. Spongy bones' trabeculae follow their bone's lines of stress and if the direction of stress changes or alters over time, the trabeculae can realign accordingly.

Osteocytes, Osteoblasts, and Osteoclasts

The cells comprising bone tissue are called osteocytes, osteoblasts, and osteoclasts:

- **Osteocytes** are found individually in spaces called lacunae within the calcified matrix of bone. They communicate with each other through small canals in the bone called canaliculi. The osteocytes in both compact and cancellous bone have a similar structure and function.

- The bone matrix is mostly formed by cells called **osteoblasts** which then sit in the matrix, transforming into osteocytes. Osteoblasts arise from mesenchymal or other undifferentiated cells. The cells are cuboidal and line the trabeculae forming in immature or developing cancellous bone.
- **Osteoclast** cells are involved in bone development and remodeling. They remove the existing mineralized bone matrix, releasing the organic and inorganic components.

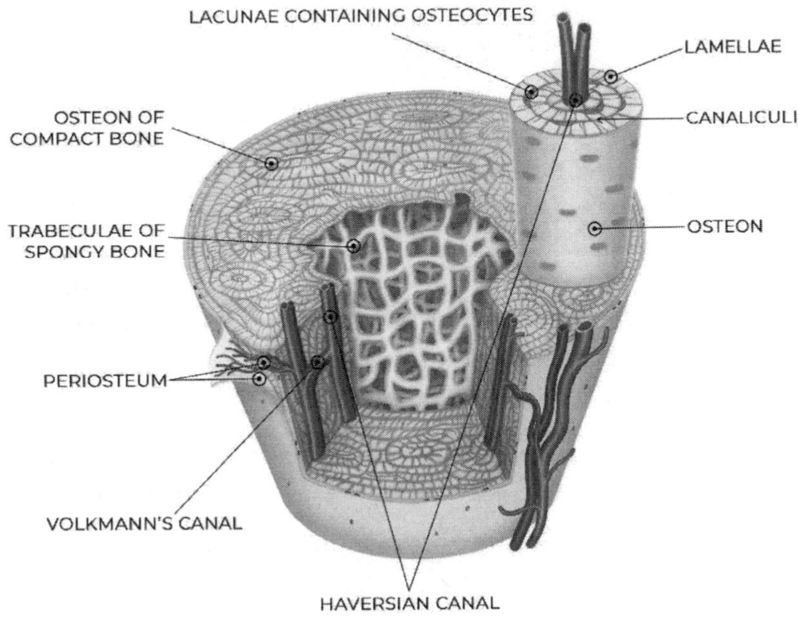

Muscular System

Muscle fibers - the specialized cells of the muscular system are contractile. Muscles are responsible for movement, whether they are attached to bones, internal organs, or blood vessels. Muscle contraction is the cause of nearly all movement in the body.

Functional Characteristics of Skeletal Muscle

The cell membrane of a muscle cell is called the sarcolemma, and it is specially structure to conduct and receive electrical impulses. The cell's sarcoplasm contains many contractile myofibrils, which relegates the nuclei and other organelles to the cell's edges.

Myofibrils, contractile units within skeletal muscle cell, consist of protein myofilaments in a regular array. With respect the direction of the muscle fiber, each myofilament runs longitudinally. There are two types of myofilaments: thin filaments and thick ones. Both bands are composed of multiple molecules of a protein - actin in the thin filaments and myosin in the thick filaments.

The thin actin filaments are attached to an elastic protein called titan at a Z-line or Z-disk. The titin extends into the myofibril, serving to anchor the position of the other bands. From one Z-line to the next defines a unit called a sarcomere.

Review Video: Muscular System
Visit mometrix.com/academy and enter code: 967216

Types of Muscle

There are three types of muscle cells in the human muscular system: skeletal, cardiac, and smooth.

- Skeletal muscles are attached to bones, enabling movement; They are under voluntary control.
- Cardiac muscle, the sole muscle type that consists of branching fibers, is striated and forms the heart.
- Smooth muscle provides movement (such as peristalsis and dilation) to the internal organs and lining of blood vessels. It is under involuntary control.

Control of movement of most muscles occurs via the nervous system, but some muscles (such as the heart) are autonomous. The human body has roughly 70,000 muscles.

Reproductive System

Function

The reproductive system of the human body is responsible solely for the production and utilization of reproductive cells, or gametes. The reproductive organs include reproductive organs, the reproductive tract, the perineal structures (external genitalia), and accessory glands and organs responsible for secreting fluids into the reproductive tract.

Male Reproductive System

The functions of the male reproductive system are to produce, maintain, and transfer **sperm** and **semen** into the female reproductive tract and to produce and secrete **male hormones**.

The external structure includes the penis, scrotum, and testes. The **penis**, which contains the **urethra**, can fill with blood and become erect, enabling the deposition of semen and sperm into the female reproductive tract during sexual intercourse. The **scrotum** is a sack of skin and smooth muscle that houses the testes and keeps the testes outside the body wall at a cooler, proper temperature for **spermatogenesis**. The **testes**, or testicles, are the male gonads, which produce sperm and testosterone.

The internal structure includes the epididymis, vas deferens, ejaculatory ducts, urethra, seminal vesicles, prostate gland, and bulbourethral glands. The **epididymis** stores the sperm as it matures. Mature sperm moves from the epididymis through the **vas deferens** to the **ejaculatory duct**. The **seminal vesicles** secrete alkaline fluids with proteins and mucus into the ejaculatory duct also. The **prostate gland** secretes a milky white fluid with proteins and enzymes as part of the semen. The **bulbourethral**, or Cowper's, glands secrete a fluid into the urethra to neutralize the acidity in the urethra, which would damage sperm.

Additionally, the hormones associated with the male reproductive system include **follicle-stimulating hormone (FSH)**, which stimulates spermatogenesis; **luteinizing hormone (LH)**, which stimulates testosterone production; and **testosterone**, which is responsible for the male sex characteristics. FSH and LH are gonadotropins, which stimulate the gonads (male testes and female ovaries). FSH and LH are gonadotropins, which stimulate the gonads (male testes and female ovaries).

Female Reproductive System

The functions of the female reproductive system are to produce **ova** (oocytes or egg cells), transfer the ova to the **fallopian tubes** for fertilization, receive the sperm from the male, and provide a protective, nourishing environment for the developing **embryo**.

The external portion of the female reproductive system includes the labia majora, labia minora, Bartholin's glands, and clitoris. The **labia majora** and the **labia minora** enclose and protect the vagina. The **Bartholin's glands** secrete a lubricating fluid. The **clitoris** contains erectile tissue and nerve endings for sensual pleasure.

The internal portion of the female reproductive system includes the ovaries, fallopian tubes, uterus, and vagina. The **ovaries**, which are the female gonads, produce the ova and secrete **estrogen** and **progesterone**. The **fallopian tubes** carry the mature egg toward the uterus. Fertilization typically occurs in the fallopian tubes. If fertilized, the egg travels to the **uterus**, where it implants in the uterine wall. The uterus protects and nourishes the developing embryo until birth. The **vagina** is a muscular tube that extends from the **cervix** of the uterus to the outside of the body. The vagina receives the semen and sperm during sexual intercourse and provides a birth canal when needed.

Review Video: Reproductive Systems
Visit mometrix.com/academy and enter code: 505450

Urinary System

Functions

The urinary system's main function is to maintain the set volume and composition of fluids of the body within the bounds of their normal limits. Because a crucial role of this system is the elimination of accumulated waste products from the body that result from cellular metabolism, it is also called the excretory system. This system maintains fluid volume at appropriate levels by regulating the water volume excreted in the urine. The urinary system also regulates the concentrations of different electrolytes circulating in body fluids and maintains the blood's pH within its normal range. It also controls the production of red blood cell by secreting the hormone erythropoietin and secretes renin to help maintain normal blood pressure.

Review Video: Urinary System
Visit mometrix.com/academy and enter code: 601053

Structures

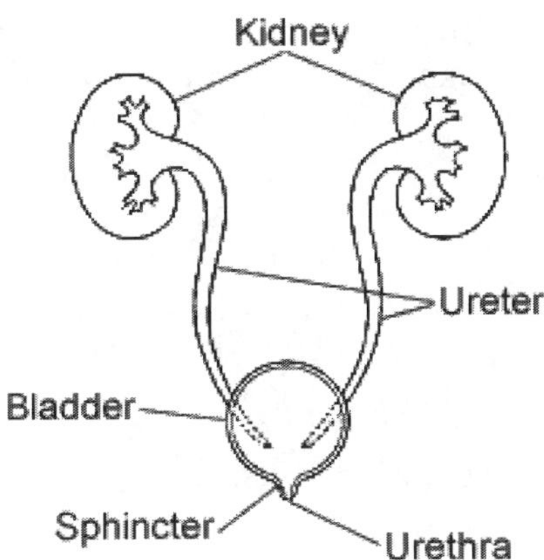

Digestive System

The digestive system consists of the digestive tract (that the ingested food passes through) and its the accessory organs, which assist in the chemical breakdown of food. The function of the digestive system is to process ingested food and beverages into smaller molecules that can be more readily absorbed and utilized by the body's cells. Food is broken down into increasingly smaller molecules until they can be until absorbed on a cellular level and the remaining waste eliminated. The digestive tract, termed the gastrointestinal (GI) tract or alimentary canal, is a long continuous tube extending from the mouth down to the anus. After the mouth, it passes through the pharynx and esophagus to the stomach, and then reaches the small and then large intestine. The mouth contains the accessory structures of the tongue and teeth, which help with the mechanical breaking up of food. The major accessory organs with a chemical role in digesting food include the salivary glands in the mouth, and the liver, gallbladder, and pancreas in the abdomen. These organs function to secrete fluids that help digest the food particles present in the digestive tract.

Review Video: Gastrointestinal System
Visit mometrix.com/academy and enter code: 378740

Functions

The six main functions of the digestive system are described below:

- Ingestion - The initial event in digestion is ingestion or taking in food through the mouth.
- Mechanical Digestion - The ingested food is in pieces that are too large for the body to use, so they must be broken down into smaller particles, increasing surface area, which various enzymes can act upon. This is the process of mechanical digestion. It begins in the mouth with mastication.
- Chemical Digestion - Via hydrolysis, the process of adding water and digestive enzymes to break down larger food molecules, chemical digestion transforms the complex and large molecules of carbohydrates, proteins, and fats into more readily absorbable molecules that can be used by the cells. Digestive enzymes increase the rate of hydrolysis, which is otherwise quite slow.
- Movement - After food is ingested and masticated, the chewed and moistened particles exit the mouth and pass through the pharynx and down the esophagus. This movement is initiated by deglutition or swallowing. In the stomach, smooth muscle contractions cause the contents to further mix together. These contractions are repetitive and occur in isolated segments of the digestive tract in succession, mixing the food with enzymes and other secretions. The rhythmic contractions that move the food particles through the alimentary canal is called peristalsis.
- Absorption - In the absorption process, the smaller molecules that result from the digestion process pass through the membranes of the cells lining in the walls of small intestine into the capillaries of blood or lymph vessels.
- Elimination - The food particles that cannot be further digested or absorbed must be eliminated. The body removes indigestible wastes in the form of feces through the anus, in the process called defecation or elimination.

Endocrine System

The endocrine system uses chemical messengers called hormones to impact metabolic activities, growth, and development. Endocrine system actions regulate the body on a slower time table than the nervous system - more on the order of minutes, hours, days, or weeks, but both systems help maintain homeostasis. The human body has two primary categories of glands: exocrine and endocrine.

Exocrine Glands - Include mammary, sweat, sebaceous, and digestive enzyme-secreting glands, which all contain ducts that secrete their product out to a surface.

Endocrine Glands - These glands lack ducts to carry their products out to a surface; thus, they are termed ductless glands. The word "endocrine" derives from the Greek words "endo," for within, and "krine," meaning to secrete or separate.

Endocrine gland secretions are called hormones and they are released directly into the blood and then travel throughout the body. Their influence is only exerted on the cells with receptor sites for that particular hormone.

Review Video: Endocrine System
Visit mometrix.com/academy and enter code: 678939

Gland Locations

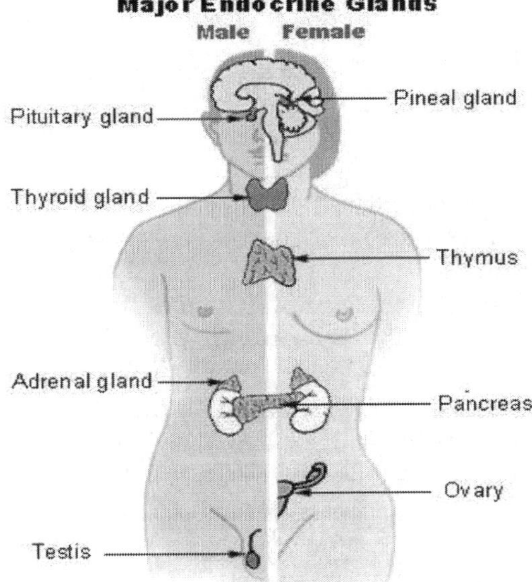

Aldosterone Levels

Aldosterone is an adrenal hormone. It has a role in the regulation of water and sodium in the kidneys. A patient must be in the upright position for at least 30 minutes prior to the collection of the specimen. Also, the test is usually performed in the chemistry department.

Growth Hormone

Growth Hormone (GH), or somatotropin, is regulated by releasing and inhibiting hormones: GHRH and GHIH (called somatostatin). GH causes musculoskeletal and tissue growth and development. It stimulates the use of amino acids for protein synthesis and lipolysis to yield fatty acids to catabolize. Sometimes, it is used to stimulate muscle growth and repair and catabolize fat. GH and somatomedins (insulin-like growth factor 1) cause a negative feedback loop. These mediators are produced by the liver, muscle cells, and other tissue. Strenuous exercise and other energy-demanding activities cause a positive feedback loop. Hypersecretion of GH in childhood causes gigantism and other forms of excessive growth. Hypersecretion in adulthood causes acromegaly, which is a condition where the bones grow excessively.

Nervous System

Functions

The nervous system is the primary controlling, communicating, and regulatory body system. It is integral in all mental activities such as thought, memory, and learning. The nervous and endocrine systems work together to regulate and maintain homeostasis. The nervous system uses receptors to help the body respond and make sense if its internal and external environment. The three primary functions of the nervous system are motor, sensory, and integrative.

CNS

The central nervous system (CNS) consists of the brain and spinal cord. Due to their vital importance, the brain and spinal cord and encased in bones for protection and located in the dorsal body cavity. The cranial vault houses the brain and the vertebral column's vertebral canal houses the spinal cord. Despite the fact that the brain and spinal cord are considered two separate organs, at the foramen magnum, they are continuous.

Review Video: What is the Function of the Nervous System
Visit mometrix.com/academy and enter code: 708428

PNS

The peripheral nervous system (PNS) consists of the nerves and ganglia. Nerves are formed from bundles of nerve fibers, similar to how muscles are formed from bundles of muscle fibers. Cranial and spinal nerves extend from the central nervous system to peripheral muscles, glands, and other structures. Ganglia are small knots or collections of nerve cell bodies located outside the central nervous system. The PNS is further subdivided into a sensory (afferent) division and a motor (efferent) division. The sensory or afferent division transmits impulses from peripheral receptors to the central nervous system. The motor or efferent division transmits impulses from the central nervous system out to peripheral muscles or organs to incite an action or effect. The motor or efferent division is further subdivided into the somatic and autonomic nervous systems. The somatic nervous system, which is also called the somatic efferent or somatomotor nervous system, functions to supply motor impulses to the body's skeletal muscles. Since these nerves afford conscious control of skeletal muscles, the system is sometimes called the voluntary nervous system. In contrast, the autonomic nervous system, which is also referred to as the visceral efferent nervous system, works to supply motor impulses to smooth and cardiac muscle, and to the epithelia of glands. It is subdivided further into two divisions: sympathetic and parasympathetic. Since the autonomic nervous system regulates functions that are involuntary or automatic, it is also called the involuntary nervous system.

Review Video: Autonomic Nervous System
Visit mometrix.com/academy and enter code: 598501

ARM NERVES

- **Musculocutaneous nerve**: Connects to all muscles in the arm's anterior section. It becomes the lateral cutaneous nerve in the interval between the biceps and brachialis, connecting to a large area of forearm skin.
- **Radial nerve**: Connects to all muscles in the arm's posterior section. With the deep brachial artery, the radial nerve descends inferolaterally around the humerus in the radial groove, further dividing into the deep and superficial branches.
    - The **deep branch** innervates the muscles.
    - The superficial branch innervates the skin but also connects to the dorsum of the hand and digits.
- **Median nerve**: Does not branch in the arm. It starts on the lateral side of the brachial artery, crossing it near the middle of the arm. It connects to most forearm flexor muscles.
- **Ulnar nerve**: Does not branch in the arm. It runs anterior to the triceps on the medial side of the brachial artery, posterior to the medial epicondyle, and medial to the olecranon, entering the forearm.

INTEGUMENTARY SYSTEM

The skin, the body's largest organ, is part of the integumentary system, which also is comprised of skin extensions like fingernails and hair. The skin has the vital role of protecting and cushioning the delicate organs of the body and providing a physical barrier to keep out foreign materials out of the body and prevent it from drying out. It also helps maintain body temperature.

Review Video: Integumentary System
Visit mometrix.com/academy and enter code: 655980

Major Structures in Skin

The following are major structures found in skin:

- Pore -- A tiny opening in the skin that serves as an outlet for sweat
- Sweat gland -- Any of the glands in the skin that secrete perspiration usually located in the dermis
- Nerve ending -- The terminal structure of an axon that does not end at a synapse
- Erector pili -- Tiny smooth muscle fibers attached to each hair follicle, which contract to make the hairs stand on end
- Hair follicle -- A hair follicle is part of the skin that grows hair by packing old cells together. Inside the follicle the sebaceous gland is found. At the end of the hair, tiny blood vessels form the root, around the root there is a white structure called a bulb, which is visible on plucked healthy hairs.
- Sebaceous gland -- A gland in the skin that opens into a hair follicle and secretes an oily substance called sebum

Epidermis Layer

As the name suggests, the epidermis, is the outermost skin layer. It has four distinct layers of epithelial tissue. The epidermis' outermost layer is the stratum corneum, which is approximately 20-30 cell layers thick. These cells are dead and completely keratinized, which forms the waterproof quality of the skin. The stratum granulosum and then the stratum lucidum are the next two layers and they are both considered to be an intermediate keratinization stage because the cells are not fully keratinized while in these layers, yet as they are pushed toward the surface when the skin grows, they become increasingly keratinized. The stratum germinativum is the deepest epidermal layer. Its cells are mitotically active, meaning they are alive and they reproduce. In this layer, the growth of skin occurs.

Dermis and Subcutaneous Layers

Dermis and subcutaneous layers of skin:

- Dermis -- The dermis is the second layer of skin, directly beneath the epidermis. Unlike the epidermis, the dermis has its own blood supply. Sweat glands are present to collect water and various wastes from the bloodstream and excrete them through pores in the epidermis. The dermis is also the site of hair roots, and it is here where the growth of hair takes place. By the time hair reaches the environment outside of the skin, it has died. The dermis also contains dense connective tissue, made of collagen fibers, which gives the skin much of its elasticity and strength.
- Subcutaneous Layer -- Beneath the dermis lays the final layer of skin, the subcutaneous layer. The most notable structures here are the large groupings of adipose tissue. The main function of the subcutaneous layer is therefore to provide a cushion for the delicate organs lying beneath the skin. It also functions to insulate the body to maintain body temperature.

Vascular System

Functions

The main functions of the vascular system include:

- Transport of cellular and chemical materials
    - Gases transported - Oxygen shuttled to the cells from the lungs and carbon dioxide (a waste product) is transported to the lungs from the cells.

  - Nutrients to cells - In addition to oxygen, other nutrients, like glucose, are transported via the circulatory system. Glucose is shuttled to the liver immediately after digestion. Glucose is used to make ATP (cellular energy) and the liver works to maintain a stable blood glucose level.
  - Cellular waste - Waste products from digestion, such as ammonia (produced from protein digestion) is transported to the liver so that it can be converted to a less toxic substance, urea, which then moves on to the kidneys, and eventually excreted in the urine.
  - Hormone transport - The vascular system transports numerous hormones that function to maintain constant internal conditions.
- Contains infection-fighting cells
- Helps stabilize body fluid pH and ionic concentration.
- Transports heat to help maintain body temperature.

Pulse and Blood Pressure

Pulse and blood pressure are defined below:

- Pulse - Blood vessel expansion and contraction caused by the blood pumped through them; calculated as the number of expansions occurring per minute.
- Blood Pressure - The force exerted in the arteries by blood as it circulates. It is divided into systolic (when the heart contracts) and diastolic (when the heart is filling) pressures

Review Video: Diastolic vs Systolic
Visit mometrix.com/academy and enter code: 898934

Anemia

Anemia refers to any condition where there is reduced oxygen carrying capacity due to a fall in hemoglobin concentration with resultant tissue hypoxia. It is defined as Hb less than 13.5g/dl in males, <11/5g/dl in females, <15g/dl in newborns to three-month-olds, and less than 11g/dl from three months to puberty. Anemia results when compensatory mechanisms fail to restore oxygen levels to meet tissue demands. The following compensatory mechanisms are seen – arteriolar dilatation, increased cardiac output, increased anaerobic metabolism, increased Hb dissociation, increased erythropoietin output, and internal redistribution of blood flow. If these compensatory mechanisms are adequate, oxygen levels are restored. If not, anemia ensues, with cardiac effects, poor exercise tolerance, lethargy, pallor, headaches, angina on effort, and claudication.

Layers of the Heart

Three layers of tissue form the heart wall. The outer layer of the heart wall is the epicardium, the middle layer is the myocardium, and the inner layer is the endocardium:

- Epicardium- the membrane that covers the outside of the heart
- Myocardium-The muscular wall of the heart, the thickest of the three layers of the heart wall, it lies between the inner layer (endocardium) and the outer layer (epicardium).
- Endocardium- membrane lining the inside surface of heart

Locations of Heart Chambers and Valves

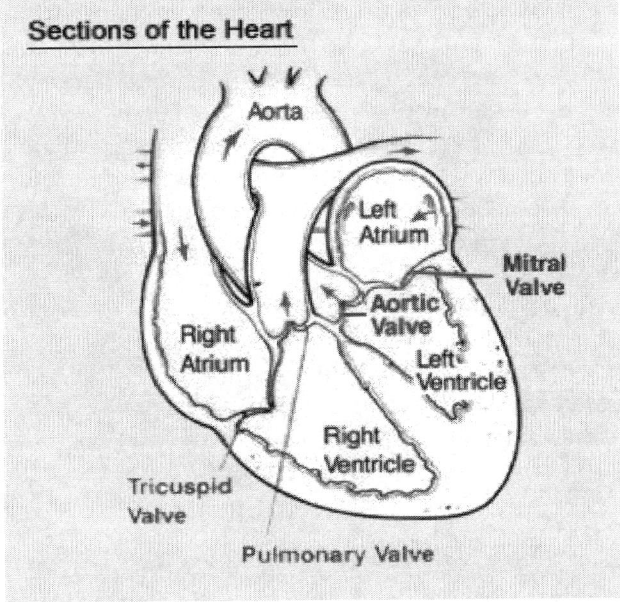

Cardiac Cycle

Ventricular Systole:

- ventricles contract
- ventricular contraction regulated by AV node
- semilunar valves (to aorta & pulmonary arteries) open
- atrioventricular valves close ("lub")

Ventricular Diastole:

- ventricles relax, atria contract
- atrial contraction regulated by SA node (pacemaker)
- semilunar valves close ("dupp")
- atrioventricular valves open

Origin of Heart Sounds

A single heartbeat lasts about one second and consists of a two-part pumping action. As blood collects in both atria (the upper chambers of the heart), the SA node (the heart's natural pacemaker) sends an electrical signal that causes atrial contraction. This contraction forces blood through the mitral and tricuspid valves into the resting ventricles (the lower chambers). This is the longer part of the two-part pumping phase, and it is termed diastole. The pumping phase's second part begins when the ventricles have filled with blood. The electrical impulses from the SA node reach the AV node and then travel to the ventricles, signaling them to contract. This phase is called systole. During ventricular contraction, the mitral and tricuspid valves close tightly to prevent the back flow of blood, but the aortic and pulmonary valves are forced open. Blood ejected from the right ventricle travels to the lungs to get oxygenated. Oxygen-rich blood leaves the left ventricle to travel to all other areas of the body. The ventricles relax, and the pulmonary and aortic valves close after blood enters the aorta and pulmonary artery. The lower pressure in the ventricles causes the tricuspid and mitral valves to open, and the cycle begins again. This system of contractions is repeated, increasing during times of exertion and decreasing while at rest.

Electrical Conduction System

The heart beats (contracts) as a result of electrical impulses from the heart muscle (the myocardium). The electrical impulse starts in the sinoatrial node (SA node), which is located in the top of the right atrium. Sometimes the SA node is referred to as the heart's "natural pacemaker." When the SA node releases the electrical signal, the atria contracts. The signal is then passed through the atrioventricular (AV) node. After checking the signal, the AV node sends it through ventricular muscle fibers, causing them to contract. The SA node sends electrical impulses at a certain rate, but your heart rate may still change depending on physical demands, stress or hormonal factors.

ECG Tracing of Cardiac Cycle

ECG tracing of a cardiac cycle is as follows:

- P wave represents the Atrial depolarization
- QRS complex represents the Ventricular depolarization
- T wave represents the ventricular repolarization

Blood Vessels

The types of blood vessels are described below:

- Arteries - blood vessels that carry blood away from the heart to the body, does not have valves
- Veins - blood vessels that carry the blood from the body back to the heart, has valves
- Capillaries – one cell thick blood vessels between arteries and veins that distribute oxygen-rich blood to the body
- Venules- the smallest veins
- Arterioles- the smallest arteries.

Layers of Blood Vessels

Wall of an artery consists of three (3) distinct layers of tunics

- Tunica intima- Composed of simple, squamous epithelium called endothelium. Rests on a connective tissue membrane that is rich in elastic and collagenous fibers.
- Tunica media- Makes up the bulk of the arterial wall. Includes smooth muscle fibers, which encircle the tube, and a thick layer of elastic connective tissue.
- Tunica adventitia - Consists chiefly of connective tissue with irregularly arranged elastic and collagenous fibers. This layer attaches the artery to the surrounding tissues. Also contains minute vessels (vasa vasorum--vessels of vessels) that give rise to capillaries and provide blood to the more external cells of the artery wall.

Smooth muscles in the walls of arteries and arterioles are innervated by the sympathetic branches of the autonomic nervous system. The Tunica media and the Tunica adventitia is much thicker in arteries.

Great Saphenous, Popliteal, Femoral, and Lesser Saphenous Veins

The locations of the great saphenous, popliteal, femoral, and lesser saphenous veins are described below:

- Great saphenous- runs the entire length of the lower extremity and is the longest vein in the body
- Popliteal- runs deep behind the knee
- Femoral- runs deep in the upper part of the leg
- Lesser saphenous- runs lateral to the ankle, up the leg and deep behind the knee

Upper Limb Arteries

Described below are the arteries of the upper limb:

- Internal thoracic - Descends posteriorly to the clavicle's sternal end and enters the thorax.
- Thyrocervical trunk - A short trunk that ascends and gives off four different branches, including the transverse and ascending cervical, and suprascapular.
- Suprascapular - Travels inferolaterally, follows the clavicle in a parallel manner, then goes posteriorly to the scapula.
- Subscapular - Descends along subscapularis muscle's lateral border to the inferior angle of the scapula.
- Thoracodorsal - Accompanies the nerve of the same name to latissimus dorsi muscle
- Deep Brachial - Accompanies the radial nerve as they pass through the humeral radial groove, then it anastomoses around the elbow joint.
- Ulnar Collateral - Anastomoses around the elbow joint.

Blood and Blood Components

Blood has numerous functions – gas transport, hemostasis, defense against disease – all of which are brought about by its various components:

- Red blood cells – oxygen transport and gas exchange
- Blood platelets and coagulation factors – coagulation and hemostasis
- Vitamin K – essential cofactor in normal hepatic synthesis of some clotting factors
- Plasmin – lyses fibrin and fibrinogen
- Antithrombin III – inhibits IXa, Xa, XIa, XIIa,
- Complement – defense against pyogenic bacteria, activation of phagocytes, clearing of immune complexes, lytic attack on cell membranes
- Lymphocytes – adaptive immune response – killing of specific microbes
- Monocytes – respond to necrotic cell material by migrating to tissues and differentiating into macrophages
- Neutrophils – phagocytosis of microbes
- Eosinophils – phagocytosis, defense against helminthic parasites, allergic reactions
- Basophils – allergic reactions

Immunoglobulins IgG and IgM

IgG is the most common class of immunoglobulin. It is also the most abundant immunoglobulin class found in blood serum and in the lymphatic system. IgG helps protect the body against a variety of detrimental agents, such as viruses, bacteria, fungi, and foreign bodies. IgM antibodies are found in the various fluids of the body. They help stimulate the production of the IgG antibodies, and IgM antibodies are some of the first antibodies that are activated to respond to antigens in the body. These antibodies play a large role in the immune response to infections in the blood.

Oxygenation and Oxidation of Hemoglobin

Oxygenation is the loose, reversible binding of Hb with O_2 molecules forming oxyHb. Hb oxygenation is the principle method of O_2 uptake from the lungs into the RBCs for transport to the tissues. Each Hb molecule has the capacity to bind four O_2 molecules since there are four heme molecules in each Hb. O_2 binds loosely with the co-ordination bonds of the iron atom in the heme and not the two positive bonds of the iron. Iron is not oxidized and oxygen can be carried to the tissues in the molecular form rather than the ionic form. Oxidation of Hb involves the conversion of the functional ferrous (Fe^{2+}) heme iron to the non-functional ferric (Fe^{3+}) form. This is called methemoglobin. This oxidized form of Hb can't bind or transport oxygen. Oxidation of Hb may occur due to exposure to toxic chemicals such as nitrites, aniline dyes and oxidative drugs.

Forces That Move Blood Through Arteries Vs. Veins

The blood flowing through the arterial system is pushed by the pressure built up by the contractions of the heart. The blood flowing through the veins relies on skeletal muscle movement to keep the valves located in the veins opening and closing to keep blood moving towards the heart and not backwards through the system.

Important Terms

Frontal (Coronal) Plane: A plane parallel to the long axis of the body and perpendicular to the sagittal plane that separates the body into front and back portions.

Sagittal Plane: A plane that divides the body into right and left halves

Transverse (Horizontal) Plane: A plane that divides the body into upper and lower sections

Extrasystole: A momentary cardiac arrhythmia manifesting as premature systole, which is also called an extra heartbeat.

Fibrillation: Inefficient and rapid heart contraction caused by disruptions to the nerve impulses.

Arrhythmia: Heart contraction rate abnormalities, which may manifest as a rate that is too slow (bradycardia) or too fast (tachycardia).

Murmur: The noise heard between normal heart sounds, due to the flow of blood through a heart valve.

Heart Rate: The number of contractions of the heart in one minute. It is measured in beats per minute (bpm). When resting, the adult human heart beats at about 70 bpm (males) and 75 bpm (females), but this rate varies between people.

Cardiac output: The volume of blood being pumped by the heart in a minute. It is equal to the heart rate multiplied by the stroke volume.

Stroke Volume: The amount of blood ejected by the ventricle of the heart with each beat, usually expressed in milliliters (ml).

Lumen: The hollow area within a blood vessel

Valves: Tissue flaps inside a vein or the heart that prevent backward flow of blood. Valves open as blood moves through them and close under the weight of blood collecting in the vein due to decreased pressure and gravity.

Patient Registration and Specimen Collection

PPT, SST, and PST

All three tubes contain thixotropic gel which is a non-reactive synthetic substance that serves as an actual physical barrier between the serum and the cellular portion of a specimen after the specimen has been centrifuged. If thixotropic gel is used in tube with EDTA, it is referred to as a plasma preparation tube (PPT.) When thixotropic gel is used in serum collection tube, the gel is referred to as serum separator thus the tube and the gel are called the serum separator tube (SST.) When thixotropic gel is used in a tube with heparin, it is called plasma separator. Thus, when thixotropic gel and heparin are in a tube; the tube is called the plasma separator tube (PST.)

Basal State

The basal state is defined at the condition of the body early in the morning while the body is at rest and has been fasting for about 12 hours. For example, a patient who at dinner at 5:00PM and wakes at 5:00AM is close to his or her body's basal state.

Disinfectant and Antiseptic

Disinfectants are used to kill possible pathogens. They are bactericidal corrosive compounds composed of chemicals. Some disinfectants are capable of killing viruses such as HIV and HBV. These are not used on humans to disinfect skin. A common disinfectant is bleach in a 1:10 dilution. Antiseptics are chemical compounds that inhibit or prevent the growth of microorganism microbes usually applied externally. Antiseptics attempt to prevent sepsis but do not necessarily kill bacteria and viruses. Antiseptics are used on human skin. Common antiseptics include70% isopropyl alcohol, betadine, and benzalkonium chloride with isopropyl alcohol being the most commonly used. Betadine is used when a sterile draw is needed.

Inversion

Inversion (the act of rotating a collection tube up and down) is carried out to mix an additive with the blood sample. Tubes without additives do not require inversions. Inversions must be done gently to thoroughly mix the additive with the sample. It's important to avoid shaking the tube or inverting too vigorously because this may result in hemolysis of the sample. If hemolysis occurs, then a number of different tests cannot be performed on the sample, including electrolyte and enzyme tests. If the inversions are done inadequately and the additive is not thoroughly mixed with the sample, microclots may develop; and these may interfere with hematology tests. If inversion of gel separation tubes does not result in thorough mixing, this may interfere with clotting. The number of inversions needed various according to the type of test and the type additive, but most additives require 8 to 10 inversions.

Patient Registration and Test Order Verification

Patient registration requires obtaining information about the patient and entering that information into the records, which are usually in an internal database. The information required includes:

- The patient's name, address, social security number, birth date, telephone number, email address (optional) and the name and telephone number of an emergency contact.
- Information about the responsible party. For example, if the patient is a child, the responsible party is generally a parent.
- Information about the policyholder's insurance, both primary and secondary. For example, patients on Medicare provide information about their Medicare coverage as well as any supplementary insurance.

Test order verification requires checking the laboratory order to ensure that it is correctly written, signed, and includes the ICD-10-CM diagnostic code for each order and that each order is appropriate for the diagnosis. For Medicare/Medicaid, verification includes determining whether the test is covered and within the appropriate time frame if it is a repeat test. Some tests may require preauthorization from insurance companies. The laboratory directory may be accessed to determine requirements for testing, such as minimum volume.

Identifying Patient Prior to Sample Collection

The first step in any blood draw or laboratory procedure for inpatients and outpatients should be to properly **identify the patient**, utilizing at least two forms of identification. Alert and responsive patients (or parents of a minor) may be asked to give their names and birthdates:

1. Introduce yourself to the patient and explain your purpose.
2. Check ID band against information provided by patient/caregiver/parent.
3. Match specimen labeling to information on ID band and label immediately with barcode labeler or permanent ink.
4. Check ankles for ID band if missing from wrists.
5. Consider only ID bands actually on the patient as valid (not on bedside stand/bed) except in special circumstances (severe burns of extremities). Verify ID with nurse in these cases.
6. If armband missing, procure armband and secure on patient before procedure.
7. Ask outpatients for picture ID and verify name and birthdate verbally if possible.
8. For emergent situations (unconscious patient in ED), check "Jane/John Doe" ID as per protocol.
9. For call reports, verify patient's name, birthdate, and ID number.

Patient Consent and Right to Refuse Treatment

Patients should give **informed consent** prior to any procedures, including laboratory tests. That is, the patient should understand the purpose, the risks, and the benefits as well as the method. Hospitalized patients sign a general consent form that covers most routine laboratory tests although some tests, such as HIV tests, may require a separate consent form. While consent may be verbal or in writing, written consent provides the most protection for the healthcare provider. **Expressed content** is consent that is given verbally or in writing. In some cases, such as in emergency care, **implied consent** is assumed, but laws vary from one state to another. Whenever a laboratory sample is obtained from a patient, the patient should first be advised the type of test and the purpose. Competent adult patients have the **right to refuse any treatment**, even if it is lifesaving. If a patient refuses a test (for example, a blood draw), the phlebotomist must immediately stop, inform the ordering healthcare provider, and document the refusal.

Initiating Patient Contact

The following are the steps in initiating patient contact:

1. Knock on door before entering patient's room, slowly open the door and ask if it is alright to enter.
2. Look for signs on door indicating special precautions that you need to take i.e. protective clothing needed
3. Identify your name and reason for entering room
4. In the event of a Physician or Member of the Clergy being in the room, it is not inappropriate to explain who you are and proceed to do the draw if the draw is STAT.
5. Ask the family to step out of the room.

Communicating with Patient During Sample Collection

The first thing a phlebotomist should do before **collecting a sample** is to make introductions to the patient, check the patient's identification (often through asking name and birthdate and checking wristband), and explain the purpose of the visit: "My name is John Doe, and I'm going to draw blood for the thyroid tests that your physician has ordered." The phlebotomist should make a point of explaining actions, "I'm going to take a look at the veins in your arms" and should ask if the patient has a preference, "Where do you prefer to have blood drawn?" if possible. If patients are quite nervous or frightened, especially young children, chatting with them briefly may help to distract them. The phlebotomist should remain professional and confident throughout the procedure and avoid making statements that may not be true, "You will barely feel this," because this violates the trust between the patient and phlebotomist.

Drawing Blood from Sleeping Patient

Drawing blood from a sleeping patient, may startle the patient and may change testing results. Also, you or the patient could be injured as the result of the patient being startled. The appropriate action to take would be to gently say the patient's name and shake the bed (never the patient) to wake them up.

Proper Patient Identification

Proper patient identification is important because it can prevent a critical error like misidentifying a patient specimen which could result in harm or death to a patient. Patient identification includes asking a patient to state their name and date of birth, and then you check the identification band and the requisition to see if they match. Verbal identification should never be relied on alone although it is important since patients can be hard of hearing, ill, or mentally incompetent and may give incorrect information. Also, check the identification band since it is possible for a patient to be wearing the wrong ID band. If there is no ID band, notify the nurse and have her confirm the patient's identity and attach an ID band before the blood is drawn. If there is any discrepancy on the ID band, information given by the patient or on the requisition, a reconciliation of the discrepancy must be made before a collection is taken. More than one patient may have the same name. Usually a name alert is placed on the chart but not in all cases.

Patient Interviewing Strategies and Techniques

Interviewing strategies and techniques include:

- Establishing rapport with the patient: Take time to make introductions and chat for a moment, especially if the patient appears anxious.
- Positioning within the patient's field of vision: Position in face-to-face position so that the patient does not have to look up or down during the interview.
- Avoiding medical jargon: Ask questions and respond in language that the patient is familiar with and explain any unclear terms used.
- Ensuring patient privacy/confidentiality: Be alert to the surroundings and make sure that questions and patient's responses remain confidential and cannot be overheard.
- Observing body language: Note nonverbal communication (eye contact, gestures, position, expressions, proxemics) for clues about the patient's emotional state and feelings.
- Asking open-ended questions: Avoid questions that can be answered with simple "yes" or "no" as much as possible.
- Allowing patient time to respond: Do not look at a watch, fidget, or appear in a hurry.
- Practicing active listening: Make eye contact, nod, respond, and pay attention when patient speaks.
- Respecting cultural differences: Avoid judgmental attitudes or comments.

Patient Preparation for Glucose Tolerance Test

A patient should eat balanced meals with 150 grams of carbohydrates for 3 days. They should refrain from eating 12 hours before the test as well as not smoking or chewing gum before or during the testing period.

Responsibility of Informing Patients of Prognosis

The phlebotomist's responsibility is not to inform a patient of his prognosis; this is the responsibility of the patient's physician. The phlebotomist may not know all the facts of the case and may give false and detrimental information to the patient. Encourage the patient to ask the physician about the prognosis.

When asked about a collection being drawn, do not discuss in detail what is being tested for since there can be various reasons why a test was ordered by the patient's physician. Respond to the patient that the physician has ordered these test as a part of the patient's medical care and that if they have any questions about them please ask the physician.

Steps in Ethical Decision Making

Steps in the ethical decision-making process:

1. Identify or determine the health problem.
2. Determine the ethical issue.
3. Obtain additional information.
4. Identify the decision maker.
5. Assess ethical and moral principles.
6. Research and consider alternative options.
7. Implement decisions as needed.
8. Assess and modify actions.

Age and Weight Requirements to Donating Blood

The donor must be between the ages of 17 and 66. The donor must weigh at least 110lbs.

Coding and Billing Procedures

Coding and billing depend on the correct choice of code when services are provided. Three different sets of codes are commonly used to bill for laboratory services:

- ICD-10-CM: Diagnostic coding comprised of 3 to 7 characters, used for both inpatients and outpatients.
- ICD-10-PCS: Procedure coding (including laboratory testing) comprised of 3-7 characters, used for inpatients only.
- HCPCSS/CPT (usually category I): Procedure coding (including laboratory testing) for outpatients.

Each laboratory test ordered must be accompanied by the correct ICD-10-CM diagnostic code. For example, if a healthcare provider orders a ferritin test for an outpatient with hereditary hemochromatosis, the ICD-10-CM code would be found under Metabolic disorders (E70-E88) as E82.110. The lab would then verify the ICD-10-CM code and apply the correct CPT code 82728 for the ferritin test. These codes are included on the charges sent to the billing department and are used to determine the correct reimbursement, based on the codes, fee schedules, and contractual agreements.

Sample Registration and Use of Laboratory Information System

Sample registration begins with patient registration, which enters identifying information about the patient into the system. If an electronic laboratory information system (LIS) is in use, then labels and barcodes for specimen tubes are generated during patient registration. When the specimen is brought to the laboratory for processing, the sample is registered as part of the existing patient registration by retrieving the patient's file, based on ID number assigned during registration and inputting information. If a LIS is not in use and laboratory records are done manually, labels and barcodes may be generated on arrival at the lab. The sample is assigned a number and the time of the collection noted as well as arrival time and the type of tube and additive. Location tracking begins, with the record indicating exactly where the sample is placed, such as the shelf, container, row, and number in a refrigerator if the sample is stored.

Nomenclature and Scheme for Prioritization of Specimen Collection and Results

Priority	Discussion
1. STAT, Med. Emergency, Immediate	Patient critical or results needed immediately. Tests include glucose, cardiac enzymes, hemoglobin and hematocrit, and electrolytes.
	Collect sample immediately and alert laboratory technicians. STAT orders from ED usually have priority over inpatient STAT orders.
2. Timed specimen	Must be obtained as close to specified time as possible to ensure meaningful results. Tests include 2-hour PP GTT, cortisol, blood cultures, cardiac enzymes. Note exact time of collection on sample.
3. ASAP (as soon as possible), Preop, and Postop	Patient is in serious but not critical condition. Tests include hemoglobin and hematocrit, electrolytes, and glucose. Preop collected before surgery to verify suitability (CBC, platelet function, hemoglobin, hematocrit, PTT, type and crossmatch) and postop to assess condition (hemoglobin, hematocrit). Some patients (preop) may be NPO.
4. Fasting	Verify fasting before collection. Tests include glucose, cholesterol, triglycerides.
5. Routine	Collect when possible but no urgency because used to monitor condition or establish diagnosis. Tests include CBC and chemistry panels.

Testing Requirements for Fasting, Medications, and Basal State

Some tests need to be carried out during a patient's **basal state**, which is the state the body is in when the patient awakens in the morning after 12 hours of fasting (no nutritional intake although water is usually allowed). In practice, patients are usually asked to fast for 8 to 12 hours, depending on the test. In addition to fasting, patients should be advised to avoiding smoking, chewing any kind of gum, or exercising as these may alter the patient's basal state and affect test results. In some cases, patients may be asked to withhold alcohol or drugs for a period of time (often the day before the test). Tests that are usually done after fasting include:

- Glucose: 8 hours.
- Triglycerides: 9 to 12 hours.
- Lipids: 9 to 12 hours.
- Renal function tests: 8 to 12 hours.
- Vitamin B-12 test: 6 to 8 hours.
- Basic/Comprehensive metabolic panels: 10 to 12 hours.
- GGT: 8 hours.
- Iron levels: 12 hours.

Minimum and Maximum Blood Volume Requirements for Common Tests

Syringes and collection tubes vary in size. Vacutainer tubes are available in multiple sizes, including pediatric, and are selected according to the usual volume needed for the specified tests. Tubes have **maximum and minimum fill** lines, and each tube specifies a draw volume, so the phlebotomist must verify this draw volume before collecting a sample, and the sample should be within 10% +/- of this draw volume if possible. Overfilling can be a problem with additives because it changes the ratio of additive to sample. Underfilling may result in a sample inadequate for testing. Typical minimum fills (but may vary according to tube size and type of tube):

- CBC and differential: 0.25 to 0.5 mL; pediatric, 1.5 mL.
- Coagulation: 2.5 m; pediatric 1.8 mL.
- Blood cultures: Varies widely, larger specimen (up to 20 mL) preferred but if <1 mL, only the aerobic tube should be filled.
- CMP: 1.2 mL.
- Electrolytes: 0.7 mL.
- Therapeutic drug levels: 0.5 mL.

Equipment for Blood Collection

Equipment needed for blood collection includes:

- Phlebotomy cart or tray to hold equipment for easy access.
- PPI, including gloves: Latex gloves should be avoided as many patients are allergic to latex, and powdered gloves pose a risk of sample contamination. Glove liners can be used for phlebotomists that are sensitive to gloves.
- Antiseptics: Isopropyl alcohol 70%, povidone iodine, and chlorhexidine gluconate are most commonly used.
- Gauze pads and bandages: Cotton balls should not be used to apply pressure on the puncture site because they may adhere to the tissue and cause bleeding when removed.
- Vein-locating devices: If necessary and available.
- Tourniquet: Non-latex are preferable. Various sizes should be available, including extra-large for obese patients and pediatric sizes. They should be flat and about 1 inch in width. May be disposable or reusable.
- Needles, syringes, tube holders, evacuated collection tubes of various types, depending on the tests to be performed.
- Sharps container: Must be available to dispose of needles.

Tourniquet

A tourniquet is used to aid in the collection of a blood specimen. The tourniquet is tied in such a way that it is easily removed above the venipuncture site. The purpose of the tourniquet is to slow down venous flow away from the puncture site and to not inhibit arterial flow to the puncture site. By doing this, the vein enlarges to make it easier to locate and puncture. A tourniquet should not be left on longer than 1 minute because this may change the composition of the blood and make testing inaccurate.

Gauge of Needle and Needle Selection

The gauge of a needle is a number that is inversely correlates to the diameter of the internal space of the needle for example the larger the needle the smaller the internal space of the needle and the smaller the number the larger the internal space of the needle. Since color-coding varies between manufactures, be careful of using this method to determine the gauge of a needle. When selecting a needle for venipuncture, there are several factors to consider which include the type of procedure, the condition and size of the patient's vein, and the equipment being used. The length of the needle used is determined by the depth of the vein. Keep in mind that the smaller the gauge the larger the bore. The 21-gauge needle is the standard needle used for routine venipuncture.

Needle Safety Devices

Needle safety devices protect the needle user's hand by having it remain behind the needle during use and by providing a barrier between the user's hand and the needle after use. Also, the needle safety devices are operable with using a one-handed technique and provide a permanent barrier around the contaminated needle.

Butterfly Needle

If a patient, such as a child or adult who is very thin with prominent veins, requires a low needle angle for venipuncture, the best choice is probably a **winged infusion ("Butterfly") set** with syringe because the syringe is not attached to the needle, so it does not get in the way, allowing a very low angle (10° to 15°) for venipuncture as the needle can be held almost parallel to the skin. Winged needles are also useful to access hand veins and scalp veins of infants. The needle (usually 23 gauge although 25 gauge may be used if vessels are extremely small) ranges from ½ to ¾ inch in length with 12 to 15 inches of tubing to which the syringe is attached. For insertion, the "wing," which are flexible, are grasped to guide the needle. For toddlers, a 23-gauge butterfly needle is often used to draw blood from the antecubital area.

Blood Collection Additives

Anticoagulant

- EDTA
- Citrates
- Heparin
- Oxalates

Antiglycolytic Agent

- Sodium fluoride
- Lithium iodoacetate

Additives Found with Colored Tube Stoppers

- Yellow – SPS and ACD
- Red (glass tube) – no additive
- Light blue – sodium citrate
- Lavender – EDTA
- Dark Green – heparin
- Gray – potassium oxalate and sodium fluoride
- Gold –silica, thixotropic gel
- Mottled red and gray - silica, thixotropic gel

Heparin

The anticoagulant heparin works by inhibiting thrombin which is required during the coagulation process. Thrombin is needed to form fibrin from fibrinogen. Thus, when thrombin is inhibited a fibrin clot is less likely to develop.

Review Video: Heparin – An Injectable Anti-Coagulant
Visit mometrix.com/academy and enter code: 127426

Inappropriate Collection Sites

The following are some variables that make a site inappropriate for selection:

1. Injuries to the skin such as burns, scars, and tattoos
2. damaged veins from repeated collections or drug use
3. Swelling (edema)
4. Hematoma (Bruising
5. Mastectomy or cancer removal including skin cancer

Selecting Equipment After Finding Collection Site

This allows you to waste less equipment if your collection site turns out to be inappropriate for the equipment you have assembled. Also, this allows for adequate drying time for the alcohol which allows for proper cleaning of the site and reduced sting from the alcohol. A site should have a minimum drying time of 30 seconds.

Proper Antiseptic Agent for Common Phlebotomy Tests

Antiseptics inhibit organisms but do not kill all of them; however, the disinfectants that are better able to kill organisms are unsafe to use of skin. A number of different antiseptics can be used for skin preparation for common phlebotomy tests:

- Isopropyl alcohol 70%: This is the most commonly used antiseptic as it is tolerated by most individuals and has good antiseptic qualities. It is usually supplied in individually wrapped pads.
- Ethyl alcohol: Generally needs to be a higher concentration and left on for a longer period of time than isopropyl alcohol.
- Povidone-iodine/Tincture of iodine: Used when higher order antisepsis is needed, such as for blood cultures. However, many patients are allergic to iodine, so this limits use.
- Benzalkonium chloride: May be used as a substitute for alcohol, such as for blood alcohol levels.
- Chlorhexidine gluconate: Used when higher order antisepsis is needed, such as for blood cultures, and recommended for IV catheter sites.

Recommended Skin Puncture Site for Older Children and Adults

The recommended site for skin puncture for this age group is the fleshy portion on the palmar surface of the distal segment of the middle or ring finger.

Reasoning Behind Wiping Away First Droplet of Blood of Skin Puncture

The first droplet of blood contains excess tissue fluid which may affect test results. Also, the alcohol residue on the skin will be wiped away with the first droplet of blood. The alcohol can hemolyze the blood specimen and keep a round droplet of blood from forming.

Preferred Method of Retrieving Blood from Child or Infant

Skin puncture is the preferred method for retrieving blood from a child or infant because children have smaller quantities of blood than adults which can lead to anemia if enough blood is drawn. Also, a child or infant may be hurt if they need to be restrained during a venipuncture. Also, infants may go into cardiac arrest if more than 10% of their blood volume is removed. If a child moves around during venipuncture, it may result in an injury to nerves, veins, and arteries.

Safest Place for Heel Puncture in Infants

NCCLS states that the safest areas for skin puncture in an infant are on the plantar surface of the hell, medial to the imaginary line extending from the middle of the big toe to the heel or lateral to an imaginary line extending from between the fourth and fifth toes to the heel.

Deep punctures of an infant's heel can lead to osteochondritis (inflammation of the bone and cartilage) and osteomyelitis (inflammation of the bone).

Appearance of Acceptable Blood Smear

A blood smear will be spread over one-half to three-fourths of the slide. There will be a gradual shift from thick to thin blood smear on the slide with the thinnest part of the slide being one blood cell thick. This thinnest part of the blood smear is sometimes referred to as the "feather." The feather part of the blood smear is the most important since the differential is performed there. In blood smears made using the two-slide method hold the slide that will smear the blood droplet at a 30-degree angle to the slide that the blood droplet was placed on.

Order of Draw

Blood collection tubes must be drawn in a specific order to avoid cross-contamination of additives between tubes. The recommended order of draw is:

1. Blood culture tube (yellow-black stopper)
2. Coagulation tube (light blue stopper). If just a routine coagulation assay is the only test ordered, then a single light blue stopper tube may be drawn. If there is a concern regarding contamination by tissue fluids or thromboplastins, then one may draw a non-additive tube first, and then the light blue stopper. This sample must be filled completely to the fill line in order to be analyzed.
3. Non-additive tube (red stopper or SST)
4. Additive tubes in this order:
    - Serum separator tube (SST; red-gray, or gold, stopper). Contains a gel separator and clot activator.
    - Sodium heparin (dark green stopper)
    - Plasma separator tube (PST; light green stopper). Contains lithium heparin anticoagulant and a gel separator.
    - EDTA (lavender stopper)
    - ACDA or ACDB (pale yellow stopper). Contains acid citrate dextrose.
    - Oxalate/fluoride (light gray stopper)

Appropriate Site for Venipuncture to Minimize Patient Risk and Optimize Outcome

The vein that is most commonly used for **venipuncture** is the median cubital, which joins the cephalic and basilic veins and is easily accessed in the antecubital space of the arm. Other veins that are sometimes used include the cephalic vein and the basilic vein. The basilic vein lies close to the median nerve and should, therefore, be the last choice. Additionally, the proximal portion of the vein lies near arteries, which can result in accidental arterial blood draw. The dorsal metacarpal veins in the hands are easily visible and accessible, but should usually be avoided in older adults because of little supporting subcutaneous tissue. The nerve most often injured with venipuncture is the median nerve because blood draws are most frequently done in the antecubital space, and the median nerve, which is the largest in the arm, passes through this area. The second most common injury is of the radial nerve, which runs near the cephalic vein on the radial side of the wrist and into the palm of the hand. Venipuncture should be avoided in the 7.5cm area above the thumb.

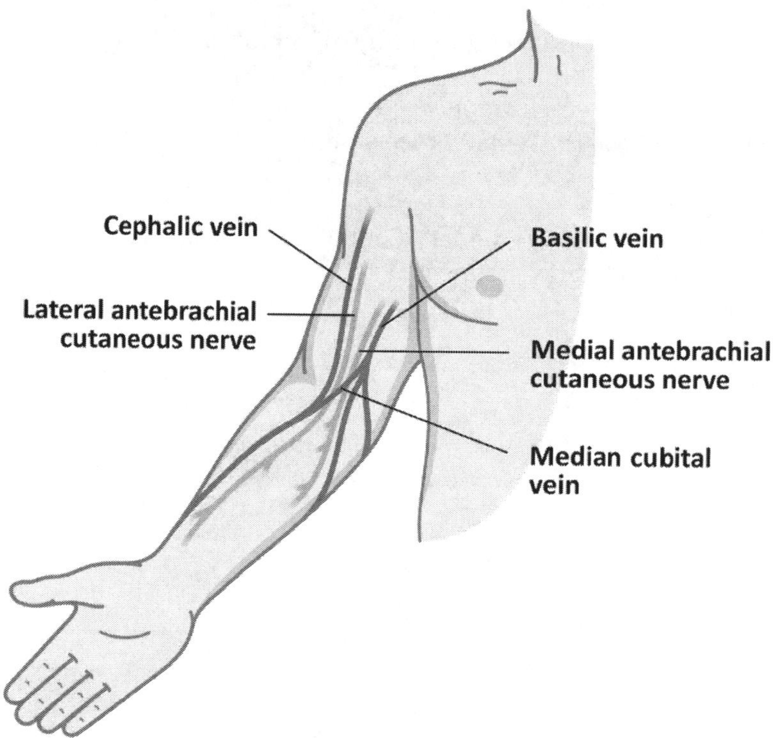

Blood Collection Procedure

Blood collection procedure:

1. Review the order, obtain proper collection tubes and equipment.
2. Explain procedure to patient and obtain 2 forms of identification (such as name and birthdate).
3. Use correct hand hygiene according to protocol.
4. Position patient in sitting position or reclining with target arm extended and supported.
5. Position tourniquet 3-4 inches above draw site (typically antecubital area) and ask patient to make a fist.
6. Identify vein, release tourniquet, and have patient open fist.
7. Apply antiseptic and air dry.
8. Prepare equipment and don gloves.
9. Apply tourniquet again and ask patient to make a fist.
10. Anchor vein and carry out blood draw.

11. Release tourniquet and have patient open fist.
12. Place a tube in the holder and twist clockwise to make sure needle pierces the stopper.
13. Fill tubes according to order of the draw to avoid cross contamination of additives: Sample in tubes with clot activators (light blue, plastic red, gold and red/gray caps) or no additives (plain red cap) are obtained before samples in tubes with anticoagulant (green [heparin], royal blue [EDTA], and lavender [EDTA]).

Clotting Time for Blood Samples

Clotting time may vary according to environmental conditions and addition of clot activators. Clotting must be fully complete before a sample is placed in the centrifuge or latent formation of fibrin may clot serum. Complete clotting usually takes between 30 and 60 minutes at temperatures of 22 to 25° C (room temperature) although this time may be prolonged in samples with a high white blood cell count or in chilled samples. Clotting is also prolonged in samples of patients on anticoagulant therapy, such as heparin or warfarin. Clot activators may be added to a sample to decrease the time needed for clotting:

- Silica particles (found in serum separator tubes) and plastic red-topped tubes require 15 to 30 minutes.
- Thrombin tubes require about 5 minutes.

Note: 5 to 6 gentle inversions of tubes with clot activators to mix it with the blood sample are required.

Blood Culture Process

Blood culture collection:

1. Verify patient identification with two identifiers.
2. Use standard precautions and venipuncture procedures, and use aseptic technique when handling equipment to avoid contamination.
3. Vigorously scrub skin with antiseptic for 30 to 60 seconds to remove skin bacteria and allow to dry.
4. Swab caps of blood culture bottles with antiseptic. Note fill line.
5. Carry out blood draw. Adults: 10-20 mL per set and pediatric patients 1-2 mL per set.
6. If multiple draws are ordered, wait 30 minutes between draws unless otherwise ordered. Take multiple draws from different sites.
7. Replace venipuncture needle with blunt fill needle and use transfer device.
8. Inject blood culture specimen into both anaerobic and aerobic bottles.
9. Mix specimen with medium in the culture bottle according to directions.
10. Label culture bottles.
11. Dispose of contaminated equipment and sharps in appropriate containers.
12. Remove gloves, sanitize hands, and transport specimen to the laboratory. Incubate and monitor as per protocol.

Minimum Requirements for Labeling Specimen

Laboratory specimens should always be **labeled** after collection with a label that is permanently attached (with adhesive). The tube or other container should never be labeled in advance, and permanent ink (generally black) should be used for any lettering:

- No pre-printed label: A label must be hand-lettered with required information, which must include the patient's full name, ID number (temporary or permanent) if available, date of birth, date and time of specimen collection, and the phlebotomist's signature or initials.
- Pre-printed label: If a label is preprinted with the patient's name and other identifying information and/or a barcode, the phlebotomist must attach the label and write the date and time on the letter and sign with signature or initials.

Any special considerations, such as "fasting" should be noted on the label as well. Before the phlebotomist leaves the patient's side, the phlebotomist should compare the label on the specimen to the patient's ID bracelet or record and the laboratory requisition to ensure they all match. Once labeled, the specimen should be placed in a biohazard bag or container for transport.

Aerobic and Anaerobic Collection for Blood Cultures

Blood collection for **blood cultures** usually involves collecting samples in two containers:

- Aerobic container: Contains air and medium to encourage growth of aerobic organisms.
- Anaerobic container: Is a vacuum and contains no air but contains a medium to encourage growth of anaerobic organisms.

Blood cultures may be done to determine the cause of fever of unknown origin and to determine if bacteremia is present. If a needle and syringe is used to collect the specimen, the anaerobic container is filled first and then the aerobic container. If a winged infusion set ("butterfly) is used, then the aerobic bottle is filled first because the tubing may contain a small amount of air. If multiple sets are ordered at the same time, each set must be obtained from a separate site although waiting 30 minutes between obtaining specimens is recommended.

Factors Impacting Ethanol Tests

Ethanol (ETHOH), commonly referred to as "blood alcohol", tests may be done for clinical or legal reasons. If carried out for legal reasons, such as to determine if a driver was under the influence of alcohol, chain of custody protocols must be followed and carefully documented. Special considerations:

- Skin antiseptics containing alcohol (isopropyl alcohol, methanol, tincture of iodine) cannot be used because they may contaminate the specimen and alter test results. Alternate skin antiseptics include povidone-iodine and aqueous benzalkonium chloride. If no alternative is available, the site should be thoroughly washed with soap and water and dried.
- Alcohol readily evaporates, so the collection tube should be completely filled and the stopper should be left on the tube until ready to perform testing.
- Testing may be done on whole blood, serum, or plasma. A glass grey top, sodium fluoride tube, with or without anticoagulant, is usually used.

Common Sites for Arterial Puncture

The radial artery is the preferred choice for arterial puncture. It is located on the thumb site of the wrist and is most commonly used. The brachial artery is second choice. It is located in the medial anterior aspect of the antecubital area near the biceps tendon insertion. Femoral artery is only used by physicians and trained ER personnel. It is usually used in emergency situations or with patients with low cardiac output.

Review Video: Arterial Punctures

Visit mometrix.com/academy and enter code: 112543

Applying Pressure to Artery After Performing Arterial Puncture

For 3 to 5 minutes directly after the needle is withdrawn from an arterial puncture, a phlebotomist should apply pressure to the puncture site. A patient should not be allowed to hold pressure since they may not hold adequate pressure for the required length of time.

Ulnar Artery

The ulnar artery provides collateral circulation for the hand. Since the radial artery is most commonly used in arterial puncture, the ulnar artery is there as a back up to provide blood to the hand if the radial artery is damaged and becomes unable to supply blood to the hand.

If Pulse Cannot Be Found or Is Faint After an Arterial Puncture

If you are unable to find a pulse after an arterial puncture or the pulse is faint, blood flow may be blocked partially or completely by a blood clot. Notify the patient's nurse or physician STAT so that circulation can begin to be restored as quickly as possible.

Allen Test

The purpose of the Allen's test is to determine the presence of collateral circulation in the hand by the ulnar artery.

Allen Test

1. Compress the radial and ulnar arteries with fingers while the patient makes a fist.
2. Patient opens hand; it should have a blanched appearance.
3. The ulnar artery is released and the patient's hand should flush with color. If this occurs, the patient has a positive Allen test and has collateral circulation of the ulnar artery.

Post Care of Venous, Arterial, and Capillary Puncture Sites

Post care for blood collection sites include:

- Venous: Place a folded gauze square over puncture site and apply manual pressure for 1 to 2 minutes until bleeding stops (longer if necessary) and then cover with pressure dressing or adhesive bandage.
- Arterial: Place a folded gauze square over the puncture site and apply manual pressure for of 3 to 5 minutes (longer with anticoagulation or coagulopathy). If bleeding, swelling, or bruising persists after initial period of manual pressure, continue pressure for an additional 2 minutes before checking again. The pressure should be maintained until all bleeding has stopped, a pressure bandage should never be used in lieu of manual pressure, and the patient should not apply pressure. Once bleeding stops, clean area with povidone iodine or chlorhexidine and check again in two minutes. Check distal pulse and notify MD if abnormal. Last, apply pressure dressing.
- Capillary: Apply pressure with a clean piece of gauze over the puncture site until bleeding stops. Because the puncture is so small, a bandage is not usually required but can be applied.

Collection of Stool Specimens

Stool specimens are obtained by placing a stool collection device in a toilet or in a bedpan. The specimen is then placed in a clean specimen container, or if for cultures, in a sterile container. Different types of containers may be used, with or without preservatives, depending on the type of tests being conducted. The sample is transferred using a tongue blade to the fill-line indicated on the container. If an additive is in the container, the sample should be shaken to mix contents. The container should be properly labeled and sealed in a biohazard bag for transport. For a stool culture, the specimen should be collected before the patient begins antibiotics. The stool specimen is placed in a sterile container or a cotton-tipped swab is inserted into the rectum and rotated to obtain a fecal sample. Then the swab is inserted into a sterile tube. Stools specimens should be processed as soon as possible or stored at 4° C if delay of more than two hours before processing.

Collection and Preservation of Extravascular Body Fluids for Chemical Analysis

Amniotic fluid	Sample collected by a physician during amniocentesis. Store in special container (protected from light) at room temperature for chromosome analysis or on ice for some chemistry tests (according to protocol).
Cerebrospinal fluid	Sample collected by physician. Collect in 3 tubes (first for culture and others for chemistry and microscopy) and store at room temperature with immediate delivery to lab. *Neisseria meningitidis* is fragile and cold sensitive, so do not chill specimen.
Gastric fluids	Sample collected during gastroscopy or from NG tube. Store in sterile container at room temperature for up to 6 hours, refrigerated for up to 7 days and frozen for up to 30 days.
Nasopharyngeal secretions.	Collected with swab or nasopharyngeal area. Place swab in tube with transport medium.
Saliva	Collected in sterile container after patient rinses mouth and waits a few minutes. Test immediately (point of care) or freeze for hormone tests to maintain stability.
Semen	Collect fresh sample from individual immediately following ejaculation into sterile container. Keep sample warm and deliver immediately for testing.
Serous fluid	Sample collected by physician, typically through thoracentesis or paracentesis. Samples labeled as pleural, peritoneal, or pericardial. Place in sterile container for C&S, EDTA tube for cell counts/smears, oxalate or fluoride tubes for chemistry tests.
Synovial fluid	Sample collected by physician through aspiration of joint. Place in ETDA or heparin tube for cell counts, smear, and crystal identification; sterile tube for C&S; and plain tube for chemistry and immunology tests.
Sputum	First morning production of sputum preferred because a larger volume is likely to be produced after sleeping. Patients should remove any dentures and rinse mouth before attempting to cough up specimen. Transport at room temperature and process immediately.
Urine	Collected in sterile container form midstream urination or catheterization. If for 24-hour quantitative testing, urine is collected in a 2L container. Store at room temperature in sterile container for 2 hours (protected from light) and then refrigerate. If both UA and C&S required, then test or refrigerate immediately.

Urine Tests

The following are some common urine tests:

1. Routine Urinalysis
2. Culture and Sensitivity – diagnosis urinary tract infection
3. Cytology Studies – presence of abnormal cells from urinary tract
4. Drug Screening – detects illegal use of drugs (prescription or illicit) and steroid, also monitors therapeutic drug use.
5. Pregnancy Test – confirms pregnancy by testing for the presence of HCG

24-Hour Urine Specimen Collection

All urine must be collected over the course of 24 hours. A large collection container is given to the patient. When a patient awakes, the first void of the morning is for the previous 24 hours and must be discarded. The next void is collected as well as the next void over the next 24 hours as well as the next morning void. Sometimes the specimen collection has to be refrigerated.

Midstream Urine Collection and Midstream Clean-Catch Urine Collection

Both involve an initial void into the toilet, interruption of urine flow, the restart of urination into a collection container, collection of a sufficient amount of specimen, and voiding of excess urine down the toilet. The clean-catch involves cleaning of the genital area, collecting urine into a sterile container and quick processing to prevent overgrowth of microorganisms, degradation of the specimen, and incorrect results.

Aspects of Urine Reviewed in Urinalysis

The following are the aspects of urine that are reviewed in a routine urinalysis:

- Physical- color, odor, transparency, specific gravity
- Chemical- looking for bacteria, blood, WBC, protein, and glucose
- Microscopic – urine components i.e. casts, cells, and crystals

Glucose Tolerance Test

The **glucose tolerance test** (GTT) is used to diagnose disorders of carbohydrate (specifically glucose) metabolism and the ability to metabolize glucose. Procedure:

1. Verify patient identification with 2 identifiers.
2. Advise patient to drink only water during the procedure and no other beverages, food, or chewing gum, and to avoid smoking.
3. Use standard precautions and venipuncture procedures.
4. Carry out blood draw (fasting) and check glucose results. Tests is usually not done if fasting glucose is >200 mg/dL.
5. Collect a fasting urine specimen if ordered.
6. Administer glucose (usually in beverage form over 5 minutes), typically 75 g for adults, 1 g/kg for children or exceptionally small adults, and 50-75 g for pregnant women.
7. Start timing and give patient schedule for collections, usually at 30 minutes, 60 minutes, 2 hours and/or 3 hours, depending on the version of the GTT ordered (usually 1-hour, 2-hour, or 3-hour).
8. Collect blood and urine (if ordered) specimens according to schedule.
9. Label specimens and transport to laboratory.

Irretrievable Specimens

Irretrievable specimens are those that require invasive procedures for collection or those that cannot be collected again and include Pap smears, meconium, placenta, cerebrospinal fluid, ascitic/pleural, peritoneal fluid, synovial fluid, and tissue samples, autopsy samples, bronchial lavage samples, urinary stone samples, bone marrow sample, pre-dialysis and pre-drug level samples, and specimens from tissue banks and eye banks. Irretrievable specimens should be labeled with at least 2 identifiers and handled carefully to avoid preanalytical, analytical, and postanalytical errors, and any waste of the sample. Protocols for each type of specimen should be followed exactly, including the time to processing, the method of transport, preservation methods, and processing procedures. For example, CSF should never be refrigerated and should be processed within 30 to 60 minutes of collection to avoid degradation of sample. Irretrievable specimens should be placed in specially labeled specimen bags for transport to the laboratory to alert personnel. The bag should be labeled with the necessary transport/storage temperature (room, iced, frozen, refrigerated).

Oropharyngeal and Nasopharyngeal Swabs

When obtaining an **oropharyngeal or nasopharyngeal swab**, the first steps are to wash the hands and don personal protective equipment, including gloves, mask, and goggles (especially important if the patient is coughing). Seat the patient upright or with the head of the bed elevated to at least 45° and head tipped back (pillows behind shoulders):

- Oropharyngeal: Depress the anterior third of tongue with tongue blade and insert swab without touching the lips, teeth, inside of cheeks, or tongue. Swab both tonsillar areas, moving the swab side to side (including any inflamed areas), and carefully remove, avoiding contact with other tissues. Insert into sterile collection tube, break off stick, secure and label.
- Nasopharyngeal: After patient blows the nose, ask the patient to occlude one nostril at a time and exhale through the nose to determine if nostrils are clear. Carefully insert the swab through the nose (or nasal speculum if necessary) to the inflamed tissue, rotate the swab in the tissue, and remove the swab without touching other nasal tissue or the speculum. Save as above.

Issues That Would Affect Way Blood Collection Should Be Performed

Many patients have allergies. These include possible allergies to adhesives, latex, and antiseptics. A patient may have a bleeding or bruising disorder that results from a genetic reason or medication that they are taking. Some patients may faint (syncope) during a procedure. It is very appropriate to recline a patient or have the lay down if they have fainted before. Some patients have a fear of needles. Some may experience nausea and vomiting from fear or an illness they have. It may be necessarily to have a trash can or spit-up container nearby for easy access. If a patient his overweight or obese then it may make a collection difficult.

Venipuncture on Dialysis Patients

Dialysis patients often have an arteriovenous shunt or fistula (usually in the forearm) created for dialysis access to filter toxins from the blood. Neither the AV shunt nor the fistula should be used to draw blood, and any blood draw should be on the opposite side. Venipuncture should be minimized in order to save veins as shunts and fistulas usually have to be periodically replaced, so if patients have advanced kidney disease and may be candidates for dialysis or already have a shunt or fistula in place, the dorsal veins of the hands should be used for blood draws and the cephalic and antecubital veins avoided. Drawing blood from foot veins should be done only if no other access is available because of increased risk of complications. When possible, capillary blood should be used. If post-dialysis blood values for BUN, sodium, and calcium are ordered, blood should be drawn within 20 seconds to 2 minutes after discontinuation of dialysis to obtain accurate results. Plasma levels of BUN increase up to 20% within 30 minutes, so timing of the blood draw is critical.

Interference with Analysis of Blood Constituents

Alcohol (70%) is the most commonly used for antiseptic skin prep, but the alcohol should dry completely prior to venipuncture because, if the alcohol contaminates the blood sample, it may result in hemolysis. Additionally, isopropanol or ethanol pads should not be used for skin prep when a blood sample is needed for alcohol testing as traces of alcohol may contaminate the sample and affect the test results. In this case, iodine is usually used, but not tincture of iodine or combined povidone-iodine with 70% ethyl alcohol because they also contain alcohol. **Iodine** preparations (2% tincture of iodine most commonly) may be used in addition to alcohol or instead of alcohol for blood draws, especially for blood culture and sensitivities, which have a high risk of contamination. Iodine should dry completely prior to venipuncture, but it should not be used if testing for iodide is being carried out as it may interfere with results

Pediatric Blood Sample Collection

For **pediatric blood draws**, care must be taken to avoid withdrawing more than 10% of the child's total blood volume. Recommended volumes are based on the child's weight:

6 to 8 lb. = 2.5 mL
9 to 10 lb. = 3.5 mL

11 to 15 lb. = 5 mL
16 to 40 lb. = 10 mL
41 to 60 lb. = 20 mL
61 to 65 lb. = 25 mL
66 to 80 lb. = 30 mL

A weight/blood draw chart should always be reviewed prior to drawing blood from an infant or child to determine how much blood can be drawn at one time and the maximum allowed within a one-month period. Blood from infants under one year of age is collected by heel stick (lateral areas), as the child's veins are generally too small for venipuncture, and fingersticks may cause bone injury. The lancet should not insert more than 2 mm to avoid damaging bone. Bandages are usually avoided in children younger than 2 years because they pose a choking hazard. Instead of a bandage, the phlebotomist should maintain pressure on a puncture or venipuncture sites, elevating the extremity for 2 to 3 minutes and checking to make sure that all bleeding has stopped. Parents should be encouraged to hold small children in a hug-hold during venipuncture and to be present to comfort older children.

Corrective Action When Blood Return Is Not Established

If **blood return** is not established with venipuncture, it may mean that the vein rolled out of the way and/or venipuncture did not occur (especially with deep veins), or the needle insertion may have been too short so that the bevel is against the vein wall and slight rotation may be sufficient to get blood return. If insertion is too long, the needle may go through the vein. The needle should always be inserted bevel up, and it can be withdrawn slightly until the bevel is just showing and slowly reinserted if necessary. However, probing and moving the needle side-to-side should not be done as it can be very painful for the patient and may damage a vessel. If moving the needle slightly does not result in blood return, then the needle should be removed and another site selected for venipuncture if possible. If the phlebotomist is unsuccessful after two attempts at venipuncture, the phlebotomist should make arrangements for a different laboratory professional to attempt the venipuncture.

Complications of Phlebotomy

Vasovagal Reaction

A **vasovagal reaction**, characterized by hypotension, diaphoresis, syncope, and nausea, may occur when a patient receives a venipuncture. If a patient complains of feeling faint and appears suddenly pale and shaky during a venipuncture (a vasovagal reaction characterized by diaphoresis and hypotension) the initial response should be to remove the needle because, if the patient faints and falls, it could dislodge the needle and result in trauma. As soon as the needle is removed, sitting patients should be assisted to put their heads low, between their legs. However, the patient is at risk of a fall injury, so the phlebotomist must support the patient. If the patient is in bed, the head of the bed should be lowered. If the patient faints and falls, an incident report must be completed and the patient examined and treated for any injury. The patient may need time to recuperate before another venipuncture is attempted.

Nausea and Vomiting

Patients may experience **nausea and vomiting** before, during, or after venipuncture because of a nervous response, vasovagal reaction, or current illness. If a patient complains of nausea before the venipuncture begins, the phlebotomist should wait until the symptoms subside unless it is an emergent situation. An emesis basin should be provided for the patient and the patient encouraged to take slow deep breaths to help the person relax. In some cases, applying a cold damp cloth to the patient's forehead may help. If the patient begins to vomit during venipuncture, the procedure should be stopped immediately and a nurse called to assist the patient. The patient should be offered tissues to wipe the mouth and water to rinse the mouth (unless NPO). Some tests may induce nausea in patients, such as the glucose tolerance test.

Clotting Deficiencies or Anticoagulant Therapy and Petechiae

Patients with **clotting deficiencies or on anticoagulant therapy**, such as warfarin or heparin, may bleed excessively after venipuncture. Patients are especially at risk for hematomas and persistent bleeding after venipuncture. Steady and prolonged pressure must be applied until bleeding stops. Elevating the arm may help to slow bleeding. A pressure dressing should not be placed instead of maintaining pressure until bleeding stops completely although a pressure dressing may then be applied and left in place for 20-30 minutes after bleeding stops as a precaution. Care must be taken to avoid excessive pressure, which may increase bruising. The phlebotomist should be aware that stroke and heart patients (such as those with atrial fibrillation) often take anticoagulants and should question medications. **Petechiae** may be a sign that a patient has a clotting deficiency, so the phlebotomist should examine the patient's skin carefully and be alert for excessive bleeding after venipuncture.

Nerve Injury and Seizures

Nerve injury can occur when the needle touches a nerve during a venipuncture, usually the result of poor site selection, improper insertion of needle, or patient movement. The pain is acute, and the patient will generally call out and complain of severe pain, tingling, or "electric shock." The phlebotomist must immediately remove the needle to prevent further damage. Once the bleeding is controlled, an ice pack applied to the site may help to decrease inflammation and pain. The phlebotomist must fill out an incident report and must follow procedures in accordance with facility protocols. Pain may persist for an extended period, and some patients may require physical therapy if nerve damage is severe.

Seizures are an uncommon complication and generally unrelated to the venipuncture; however, if a seizure occurs, the phlebotomist should immediately discontinue the venipuncture, apply pressure to the insertion site without restraining the patient and call for help. The phlebotomist should try to prevent the patient from harm. If the patient is seated, the patient may need to be eased onto the floor with assistance.

Edema and Post-Mastectomy

Blood should not be drawn from edematous tissue because the **edema** may result in the blood diluted with tissue fluids. Edema is often most pronounced in the hands and feet, but arms may be edematous as well. With generalized edema, the phlebotomist should try to find the least edematous site for venipuncture, should apply gentle pressure to the site to displace the fluid if possible, and should note on the label that edema was present.

Blood generally should not be obtained on the side of a **mastectomy**, regardless of the length of time since surgery, because the circulation may be impaired and edema may be present. Any degree of lymphedema may alter the results of the blood tests, and the patient is at increased risk of infection from venipuncture. If no other site is available, then a physician's order should be obtained regarding use of this site. With double mastectomy, especially if any degree of lymphedema is evident, alternate sites, such as feet and legs may need to be considered. If possible, a sample may be obtained through capillary puncture for lymphedema, but for generalized edema, the sample will be diluted.

Pre-Existing Intravenous Line

Blood samples should not be obtained from an existing **intravenous line** because the sample may be contaminated with IV fluids/drugs or diluted. Additionally, the sample is more likely to undergo hemolysis and need to be discarded. Blood should also not be drawn from the same side as an IV line. If blood must be drawn from an arm that has an intravenous line in place, the IV should be clamped for at least two minutes before the specimen is collected to allow the IV fluid to enter the circulation and reduce the dilution of the blood sample. It is preferable to do the venipuncture at least 5 inches distal to the IV insertion site when possible with the tourniquet also applied distal to the IV insertion site. The site (proximal or distal) in relation to the IV should be documented.

Hematoma

During a venipuncture, if the needle goes through the vein and a **hematoma** begins to rapidly develop, the next step is to remove the needle and tourniquet and apply pressure to prevent further loss of blood into the tissue. A hematoma may also form if the needle only partially penetrates the vessel wall, allowing blood to leak into the tissue. If blood flow stops and a small hematoma begins to form, the needle's bevel may be up against a vessel wall, so rotating it slightly may stop the leak and allow blood to flow into the collection tube. If a very small hematoma is evident during venipuncture, the best initial response is to observe the site and complete the venipuncture. If, however, the hematoma is large or expanding, then the phlebotomist should remove the needle, elevate the arm above the level of the heart, and apply pressure until the bleeding stops. Small hematomas are fairly common, especially in older adults whose veins may be friable and those taking anticoagulants and certain other drugs.

Allergies

Patients should be questioned about **allergies** prior to having blood withdrawn. Common allergies that may pose a problem include:

- Latex: Reactions range from mild to severe anaphylaxis, and latex allergies are increasingly common for those with frequent contact with healthcare, especially those with multiple surgeries and those with spina bifida. The phlebotomist should avoid taking any latex items, such as tourniquets and bandaging supplies, near the patient with a severe allergy and should generally replace latex items with non-latex for all patients.
- Iodine: Patients may be allergic to any skin antiseptic, but allergy to iodine is most common. Patients who report being allergic to fish are also at risk for iodine allergy. Alternate antiseptics should be used in place of antiseptics with iodine.
- Adhesive: Some patients are allergic to adhesive, which may cause itching and rash. Some types of tape, such as paper tape, are better tolerated but may still cause a problem for some patients. Stretch bandaging materials (such as Coban®) may be used to secure a dressing.

Medications and Recent Surgery

Medications that pose a particular concern with phlebotomy are those that interfere with clotting mechanisms:

- Platelet inhibitors, such as aspirin, clopidogrel (Plavix®), and abciximab (ReoPro®).
- Anticoagulants include injectable drugs such as heparin, argatroban, and bivalirudin and Oral anticoagulants, such as warfarin (Coumadin®), rivaroxaban (Xarelto®) and Dabigatran (Pradaxa®).

All of these drugs increase the risk of bleeding, so multiple venipunctures should be avoided when possible. Care must be taken to apply pressure until all bleeding stops, and a compression dressing may then be left in place for at least 20 minutes to ensure no recurrence of bleeding.

Recent surgery may pose a risk of complications, depending on the type of surgery and the medications given to the patient after surgery. Blood should not be drawn from an arm that has recently undergone any type of surgical procedure or the arm on the side of a mastectomy or any surgery that might interfere with blood flow or lymph flow.

Dehydration and Chemotherapy

Dehydration may occur in patients with severe nausea and vomiting and/or diarrhea and those with inadequate fluid intake for body needs. Dehydration results in decreased cardiac output and blood volume, so blood vessels constrict, making it difficult to access the veins and resulting in hemoconcentration that affects test results. If possible, the blood draw should be delayed until the patient is more hydrated; but, if it is necessary to draw blood, a warm compress may help to dilate the vessels slightly. A smaller gauge needle or a winged infusion set may also be necessary. The label should indicate the patient is dehydrated and the physician notified.

Patients on **chemotherapy** often have central lines, such as ports or PICC lines and these may, at times, be used to withdraw samples, but phlebotomists are generally prohibited from drawing specimens through central lines. Veins may be fragile and collapse easily, so a smaller gauge needle or winged infusion set may be necessary. Warming the site may help to make the veins more visible. Edema may obscure veins, and prolonged bleeding may occur because of coagulopathy.

Geriatrics

Drawing blood from **geriatric patients** poses a number of challenges:

- Disabilities: Patients may be hard of hearing and/or have difficulty speaking, interfering with communication with the patient. The phlebotomist should speak clearly but avoid shouting and allow the patient extra time to respond or indicate comprehension. For patients with vision impairment, the phlebotomist should guide the patient and explain all actions verbally. If a patient has dementia, the phlebotomist should speak in simple sentences and reassure the patient, asking for help if the patient is hostile or combative. Physical disabilities (arthritis, neuromuscular diseases, contractures) may limit mobility.
- Aging: Loose skin and loss of muscle tissue may make it difficult to anchor a vein, and veins may be sclerosed or rolling, so careful anchoring of the vein is necessary. Scarred, sclerosed veins should be avoided. Circulation may be impaired (especially with diabetic patients), and medications (such as anticoagulants) may increase bleeding or interfere with test results. Prolonged pressure may need to be applied to puncture sites, and heavy adhesives may tear skin.

Obesity

Obesity can pose a problem for venipuncture because the patient's veins may be deep and not visible or palpable. The median cubital vein in the antecubital area should be examined first as it may be palpable between folds of tissue. However, with obese patients, the cephalic vein is often easier to palpate than the median cubital vein. Rotating the hand into prone position (palm down) may make the cephalic vein more palpable. In some cases, a longer needle may be necessary for venipuncture. If there is no or little fat pad on the top of the hand, then the hand veins may be used for venipuncture. Tourniquets may be difficult to position as they tend to roll and twist. An extra-large tourniquet or Velcro closure strap should be used if possible but, if not available, using two tourniquets, one on top of the other, may help keep the tourniquet from twisting. Patients may know from past experience which access site is best, so the phlebotomist should ask the patient directly.

Risks to Patients if Complications or Errors Occur in Blood Collection

Some of the risks to patients if a complication or error results from blood collection are as follows:

1. Arterial puncture
2. Anemia resulting from the procedure
3. Infection
4. Hematoma (bruising) of the venipuncture site
5. Damage to a nerve if punctured
6. Vein damage
7. Pain

Hematoma

Described below is how a hematoma can result from errors in phlebotomy techniques:

1. inadequate pressure to the collection site after a blood draw
2. blood leaking through the back of a vein that was pierced
3. blood leaking from a partial pierced vein
4. an artery is pierced

AFP

AFP is alpha-fetoprotein. Normally it is found in the human fetus, but abnormal levels of AFP may indicate a neural tube defect in an infant or other fetal developmental problems. The test is performed on maternal serum. If results are abnormal, a test on the amniotic fluid will be used to confirm results.

Endocrine System Tests

Endocrine tests include:

- Aldosterone: Mineralocorticoid produced by adrenal glands in response to increased potassium, decreased sodium, or decreased blood volume. Helps to regulate sodium and potassium levels. Specimen collected with plain red top tube and tested on serum (refrigerate after centrifugation). "Up-right" sample should be obtained after patient in sitting position for at least 30 minutes.
- Renin: Enzymatic hormone secreted by the kidneys in response to sodium depletion. Tested to determine cause of hypertension. Test usually conducted along with aldosterone level. Specimen collected in lavender-topped EDTA or pink-topped EDTA tubes and tests conducted on plasma.
- Cortisol: Primary glucocorticoid secreted by adrenal glands. Stimulates gluconeogenesis, serves as insulin antagonist, suppresses inflammatory response, and mobilizes proteins and fats. Test assesses adrenal function and to diagnose Cushing's disease and Addison's disease. Specimen collected for serum test in red or red/gray topped tube and for plasma tests in green-topped heparin tube. If serial tests are done, the same type of tube should be used for all tests. Time of draw must be correctly notes. Tests are often done at 8 AM and 4 PM.
- Glucagon: Hormone produced in the pancreas and excreted by kidneys, increases amount of glucose and fat in the blood. Specimen collected in chilled lavender-topped EDTA tube and test conducted on plasma. Specimen must be tightly capped and placed in ice slurry for transport.
- Insulin: Hormone produced in the beta cells of the pancreas, regulates metabolism of proteins, fats, and carbohydrates, controls production and storage of glucose. Test done to determine the amount of insulin secreted in response to glucose and may include administration of standardized dose of glucose at fixed time periods. Specimen is collected in red-topped tube, and test conducted on serum.
- Erythropoietin (EPO): Hormone produced in the kidney promotes red cell production. Test assesses cause of anemia and/or kidney function. Specimen collected in red, gold, or red/gray top tube, and test conducted on serum. Phlebotomy may increase levels of EPO.

EDTA

Ethylenediaminetetraacetic acid (EDTA) is a potassium-based or sodium-based anticoagulant used in blood collection tubes (usually lavender and pink) to prevent clotting of the whole blood specimens (CBC and blood component tests) and to save specimens for blood bank testing. EDTA binds calcium to prevent clotting and preserves cell morphology and prevents the aggregation of platelets. The tube should be filled to the specified level and the correct tube size selected for the necessary volume. Eight to 10 inversions are needed immediately after sample collection in order to thoroughly mix EDTA with the blood because failure to adequately mix them can result in formation of microclots or aggregated platelets. EDTA may be in liquid form (K3EDTA) or spray-dried (K2EDTA), but the liquid form may dilute the sample and alter test results (1-2% decrease). EDTA tube with blood sample should be placed in a refrigerator while awaiting processing. The timing and storage requirements vary according to the type of test. For example, red blood cells count remains stable for up to 72 hours under refrigeration, but white blood cell counts are less stable.

Collection Tube Tests, Additives, Specimen Type, Number of Inversions, and Department

Black, Dark Blue, and Light Blue

Collection tube	Black	Blue (dark)	Blue (light)
Tests	ESR	Toxicology, trace metals, nutritional analysis	Coagulation
Additives	Sodium citrate	EDTA, heparin, or none	Sodium citrate
Specimen	Whole blood	Plasma or serum	Plasma
Inversions	0	Heparin or EDTA—8-10. No additive-0.	3-4
Department	Hematology	Hematology	Hematology
Notes	Do not invert. Fill tube completely.	Verify additive before proceeding.	Fill tube completely.

Gold/Tiger-Top/Red-Gray, Gray or Light Gray, Dark Green

Collection tube	Gold, tiger-top, red-gray	Gray, Light gray	Green (dark)
Tests	Blood chemistries, serology, immunology	Lactic acid, GTT, FBS, blood alcohol	Blood chemistry, ammonia, electrolytes, ABG
Additives	Clot activator and/or thixotropic gel	Iodoacetate, sodium fluoride, and/or potassium oxalate or heparin or EDTA	Heparin (sodium)
Specimen	Serum	Plasma	Plasma or whole blood
Inversions	5-6	8-10	8-10
Department	Chemistry	Chemistry	Chemistry
Notes	AKA serum separator tube	May need to be placed on ice.	STAT test

Light Green or Gray/Green, Lavender, and Orange or Yellow-Gray

Collection tube	Light Green, Gray/Green	Lavender	Orange, Yellow-gray
Tests	Potassium, chemistry tests	CBC, molecular tests	Chemistry tests
Additives	Heparin (lithium), thixotropic gel	EDTA	Thrombin
Specimen	Plasma	Whole blood	Serum
Inversions	8-10	8-10	8-10
Department	Chemistry	Hematology	Chemistry
Notes		Most common test	STAT test

PINK, RED (GLASS), RED (PLASTIC)

Collection tube	Pink	Red (glass)	Red (plastic)
Tests	Hematology, Typing and screening	Chemistry, serology, immunology, crossmatch (for blood bank)	Chemistry, serology
Additives	EDTA	None	Clot activators
Specimen	Whole blood	Serum	Serum
Inversions	8-10	0	0
Department	Blood bank	Chemistry	Chemistry
Notes	Do not confuse pink and lavender tubes.	Specimen must rest 30 minutes. Do not confuse with plastic red tube.	Specimen must rest 30 minutes. Do not confuse with glass red tube.

TAN, STERILE YELLOW, NON-STERILE YELLOW

Collection tube	Tan	Yellow (sterile)	Yellow (non-sterile)
Tests	Lead analysis	Blood culture	HLA, paternity test, tissue typing
Additives	K2 or EDTA	SPS	Acid citrate dextrose (ACD)
Specimen	Plasma	Whole blood	Whole blood
Inversions	8-10	8-10	8-10
Department	Chemistry	Microbiology	Chemistry
Notes		Do not confuse with nonsterile yellow tube.	Do not confuse with sterile yellow tube.

IMPORTANT TERMS

Malpractice: A lawsuit raised against a professional for injury or loss resulting from negligence on the part of the professional in rendering services.

Negligence: Failure to perform or act with the prudence expected by a reasonable person in the same circumstance.

Hemoconcentration: Increased concentration of components found in the blood because of decrease in the fluid portion of the blood.

Sclerosed: Refers to veins that are hard and cord-like from scarring or irritation, rendering them difficult to puncture and impairing blood flow at the sclerosed site.

PKU: Abbreviation for phenylketonuria, an inherited disorder of amino acid metabolism in which the body cannot metabolize phenylalanine (found in proteins) so it builds up in the body and can damage the brain.

Lipemia: Abnormal amount of lipids (fats) in the blood.

Petechiae: Small, sometimes pinpoint, reddish-purple hemorrhagic lesions on the skin, associated with high fever and thrombocytopenia.

DNR: Do not resuscitate. No codes should be called for this patient and no heroic measures should be taken to revive patient if the patient stops breathing.

NPO: From the Latin phrase nil per os meaning nothing by mouth. Patients are not allowed food or drink including water. This restriction is usually placed on a patient before and after a procedure.

STAT: From the Latin word statim means immediately. It describes the need for a specimen or test to be done immediately in response to critical situations with the possibility of the test results preventing a patient's death.

ASAP: As soon as possible, this is used if the results are needed soon but not to prevent the patient from dying

Fasting: When a person refrains from eating or drinking anything before a procedure, sometimes water is allowed on a fast

Bevel: Slanted tip of a needle used to puncture the skin and vein without removing a piece of the vein.

Plunger: The part of the syringe that when pulled on creates a vacuum allowing the barrel of the syringe to be filled with fluid or air.

Hub: End of a needle that attaches to the blood collection device i.e. syringe or tube holder

Shaft: The hollow round long cylinder-shaped part of a needle

Sharps container: An easily sealed, rigid, leak-proof, puncture-resistant, disposable box with a locking lid in which used needles and sharp materials are disposed.

Blood smear: Blood layer on a glass slide made from a drop of blood

Capillary blood gases: Blood gases retrieved from an arterialized skin puncture

Interstitial fluid: Liquid found between cells

Intracellular fluid: Liquid found within cell membranes

Specimen Preparation and Processing

SOP for Laboratories

Each laboratory should draw up a **standard operating procedure document (SOP)** that outlines all the processes and procedures associated with reception of a sample and processing, including:

- Specimen collection processes: PPE, patient identification, collection tubes, collecting procedures, need for special handling, labeling, transporting specimens, criteria for rejecting inadequate sample, protocols for adverse reactions.
- Chain of custody: Labeling, storing, packing, and transporting.
- Sample reception: Specimen identification, logging, specimen condition, specimen accountability, retention times.
- Rejection criteria: Incorrect collection tube, leaking tube, incorrect labeling, incorrect sample for test, volume inadequate, order unverified, mismatch between order and labeling.
- Delivery (from reception to processing); Process for delivery to correct department, specimen retention policies.
- Processing: Procedures for testing, accountability standards, storage and retention policies.
- Reporting: Methods of reporting and timeframes.

Issues Related to Add-On Requests

Add-on requests are tests ordered on the same sample after the original laboratory test is completed. Add-on requests, as all laboratory orders, must be received in writing, paper or electronic. The add-on requests may be part of the original order indicating that if a test result is abnormal, then one or more additional tests should be carried out. The add-on test may also be ordered once the original test results are received. Add-on requests should indicate the sample that the add-on applies to. Some considerations:

- Length of time the specimens are saved.
- Storage: refrigerated, room temperature, frozen.
- Specimen viability.
- Adequacy of sample.

For example, if a hematology sample is kept at room temperature, some tests, such as CBC, can be carried out within 24 hours of collection time. Some tests (such as the reticulocyte count) can be carried out within 24 hours if the sample is refrigerated. Other tests must be conducted within 1 to 12 hours of collection time, depending on the type of specimen. Some add-on tests should be avoided because the results may be inaccurate, including glucose, potassium, and bilirubin.

Aliquot

When a specimen is collected, it may need to be divided to run several tests on it. An aliquot is a fraction of the specimen. Each aliquot has its own tube for testing and is label with the same information as the original specimen.

Reasons Specimens May Be Rejected for Analysis

Some reasons why a specimen may be rejected for testing include incorrect or incomplete identification, collected in an expired tube, inadequate amount of specimen collected (QNS, quantity not sufficient), and collection in an incorrect tube.

Importance of Proper Handling of Specimen Before Analysis

46 to 68% of lab errors result from improper handling of a specimen before it was analyzed. For example, if an anticoagulant tube is improperly mixed, it may result in microclots forming. If a tube is shaken too hard hemolysis of the specimen may occur. If a specimen is not cooled properly then metabolic processes may continue after collection which may skew test results.

Chain-of-Custody Specimens

Chain-of-custom specimens are those for which a laboratory has established a documented record that shows every consecutive person in contact with the specimen from the time of collection through transfer and to the time of disposition (both internal and external contact and including date, time, and signature) and ensures that no tampering with the specimen has occurred in order to meet legal requirements. The document must outline provisions for securing long-term storage. Chain-of-custom specimens may include specimens for blood alcohol, drugs, or crime scene testing, often including blood, urine and DNA testing. The chain-of-custom SOP may include labeling requirements, temperature requirements, expected timeline, packing, and transporting specifications. The person from whom the sample is obtained must be clearly identified as well as the name of the collector and the time, date, and location of obtaining the sample. Containers in which a sample is transported should be secured with custody tape.

Interpersonal Communication with Non-Laboratory Personnel

Interpersonal communication skills are essential for the laboratory professional, who must interact with a variety of non-laboratory personnel in the work environment. Elements of effective communication include:

- Showing respect and consideration to others in all communications.
- Recognizing each individual's scope of practice and responsibilities toward the patient.
- Being an active listener, paying attention and asking clarifying questions as necessary.
- Sharing important information with the appropriate personnel.
- Asking questions when in need of more information about a patient.
- Ensuring that information is shared accurately.
- Providing timely communication.
- Discussing special needs of patients in relation to collection of a sample and processing.
- Communicating any problems encountered with collection or processing with the appropriate personnel.
- Discussing timing issues related to sample collection, such as STAT orders or collection that must be done at a specific time.
- Scheduling collection to avoid interrupting other patient care activities when possible.

Assessing Specimen Quality

Issues of **specimen quality** include:

- Hemolysis: Pink discoloration of plasma and serum because of the presence of damaged red blood cells and hemoglobin. May result from abnormal condition, such as hemolytic anemia, or from incorrect handling. Hemolyzed samples may interfere with some tests (electrolytes, iron, enzymes), so the sample will likely need to be redrawn.
- Quantity not sufficient (QNS): May occur if the volume of blood in the collection tube is insufficient for testing or if the blood-anticoagulant ratio is incorrect. Short draws may be sufficient for some tests if the specimen is not hemolyzed. With QNS, the usual solution is to obtain another specimen.

- Clotting: May result from maintaining a sample in a syringe with no anticoagulant for too long before transferring to a tube, carrying out a very slow draw with a syringe that allows clotting to begin, and failing to adequately mix the sample with the anticoagulant. If clotting occurs, a new sample must be obtained.
- Incorrect specimen type: If the incorrect specimen type is obtained or a specimen is obtained in a collection tube with the wrong additive, then another specimen must be obtained in order to carry out the intended tests.

Procedures to Prevent Hemolysis

Hemolysis, rupture of red blood cells, is the most common reason laboratory specimens must be redrawn. Steps to preventing hemolysis include:

1. Utilize large gauge (20 to 22) needle for blood draws for large veins, such as the antecubital.
2. Warm draw site to improve blood flow.
3. Keep tourniquet on no longer than 60 seconds.
4. Air-dry alcohol applied to skin prior to blood draw.
5. Utilize partial vacuum tubes if possible.
6. Avoid milking veins or capillary puncture sites.
7. Avoid excessive pressure when pulling or pushing on plunger.
8. Avoid blood draws from catheters or vascular access devices.
9. Ensure volume in tubes with anticoagulant is sufficient.
10. Avoid vigorous mixing or shaking of specimens.
11. Invert tubes with clot activator 5 times, with anticoagulant 8 to 10 times, and with sodium citrate 3 to 4 times (coagulation tests).
12. Store and transport specimens at appropriate temperature.
13. Use appropriate centrifugal speed and duration for processing samples that have clotted completely.

Laboratory Results

Information that must be included on the **laboratory results** includes the name, address, and contact information for the lab, the patient's name, birthdate, gender, and ID number (if one is assigned) and the name of the requesting provider. The results must include the date and time the specimen was collected and the date and time each test result was verified. The tests should be listed along with the value, units, and reference ranges with some indication of abnormal values, such a high (H) or low (L), abnormal (A), critical high (CH) or critical low (CL). The lab results should be separated by type, such as chemistry panels and hematology panels. Laboratory results may be distributed to ordering providers in a number of different ways:

- Paper: May be delivered by courier, placed in physician's hospital mailbox, or mailed.
- Telephone: Results may be transmitted by phone even when paper or other type of report is given to ensure that the ordering provider receives the information in a timely manner, especially when there are abnormal results.
- Messaging/Email/Electronic: Must be delivered over secure lines so that confidentiality is not compromised. Reports may be sent automatically. If patients can access through a patient portal, the ordering provider may need to access the report first and indicate it can be released to the patient, depending on how the system is set up.

Specimen Assessment and Rejection Criteria

Specimens must be obtained following established protocols and in the proper tube or container with the correct additive, such as sodium citrate in a blood specimen. The specimen must be stored and/or transported in a manner appropriate to the type of specimen. **Rejection criteria** may vary according to the type of specimen and test, and specimens are generally not discarded until the ordering healthcare provider is notified. Rejection criteria may include:

- Incorrect tube or container.
- Incorrect or missing requisition/order.
- Specimen size insufficient for testing.
- Hemolysis evident.
- Specimen not correctly labeled.
- Tube/container leaking or contaminated with body fluids. (Note: critical specimens may be salvaged after tube/container thoroughly cleansed with 10% hypochlorite [bleach] solution.)
- Specimen contained in syringe with attached needle.
- Date/Collection time not noted on specimen.
- Specimen too old for testing.
- Specimen improperly stored/transported.

Aliquoting a Sample

Aliquoting a sample is done to withdraw serum or plasma from whole blood and/or to divide one sample into multiple aliquots for different tests. The individual must apply PPI, including gloves and goggles, and prepare aliquot tubes with appropriate labels. Aliquoting is done after centrifugation with anticoagulated tubes aliquoted into plasma specimens and coagulated tube aliquoted into serum specimens. It's necessary to place the centrifuged tubes into a rack and to avoid inverting the sample after centrifugation because this will cause remixing. A disposable pipette (never use a mouth pipette) is used to transfer each aliquot, starting from the top of the sample and working downward toward the point of separation. The aliquots are transferred to labeled tubes. As soon as an aliquot tube is filled, it must be capped. Aliquoted samples must be carefully labeled because serum and plasma are indistinguishable once they are aliquoted. Some other types of samples, such as saliva, must be mixed using a vortex mixer prior to aliquoting to ensure the sample is homogenous. Aliquots should be placed promptly in the appropriate storage, such as the refrigerator or -20° or -80° C freezer.

Settling of Blood in Anticoagulant Tubes

Describe below is how blood in an anticoagulant tube will settle after being centrifuged or being allowed to settle:

- The top layer will be the plasma.
- The next thin layer is the buffy coat made of white blood cells and platelets.
- The bottom layer is red blood cells.

Properly Centrifuging a Specimen

The centrifuge needs to be evenly balanced with tubes of equal size and volume across from one another. Stoppers should always be in place to prevent aerosol. Also, be sure to allow complete clotting before centrifuging the specimen. If a specimen is not completely clotted before centrifuging then it may result in latent fibrin formations clotting the serum. Never centrifuge a specimen twice.

Chilling a Specimen

The most appropriate way to chill a specimen is to immerse it into an ice and water slush. Ice cubes alone will not allow for adequate cooling of the specimen, and where the ice cubes touch the specimen may freeze it resulting in possible hemolysis or breakdown of the analyte.

Inverting a Tube

A tube should be inverted if it contains an additive and if the manufacturer's instructions require for it to be inverted. If the tube in a nonadditive tube then it does not have to be inverted. An additive tube usually is inverted between three and eight times to properly mix the additive with the blood.

Preventing Aerosol Formation When Stopper Has No Safety Feature to Prevent Aerosol

The stopper should be covered with 4x4-inch gauze and placed behind a safety shield to ensure the aerosol is not inhaled. Proper protective clothing should be worn as well. A safety stopper removal device may also be used.

Temperature Requirements for Specimens

Specimen storage is often at room **temperature**, which is generally based on the range found in temperature-controlled buildings: 20° C to 25° C. Blood bank and laboratory specimen refrigerators are maintained between 2° C and 4° C. Freezers are maintained at -20° C with some specialty freezers at -80° C. Incubators usually provide for a range of temperatures (5° C to 70° C) with much incubation done at 37° C (body temperature). Samples may remain viable for different periods of time, depending on how they are stored. Some serum and plasma samples must be frozen prior to shipping. Temperature requirements depend on the types of specimen and the test.

Transport with heat block at 37° C	Transport in ice slurry and refrigerate (freezing may cause hemolysis)
Cryoglobulins, cryofibrinogen, and cold agglutinin.	ACTH, acetone, ACE, ammonia, blood gases, catecholamines, FFA, gastrin, glucagon, homocysteine, lactic acid, PTH, blood pH, pyruvate, renin.

Shipping Patient Samples

Note that personnel responsible for **shipping** of specimens must have been appropriately trained and understand possible hazards, according to regulations by the Department of Transportation, International Civil Aviation Organization, and CDC. Frozen serum and plasma must be shipped in plastic tubes (not glass) with screw-on caps for security and labeled with 2 patient identifiers. The tubes are wrapped in absorbent material in case of leakage and secured in a container that is airtight (such as Saf-T-Pak®) and labeled "biohazard," placed inside of a Styrofoam container for insulation with dry ice and in a clearly labeled secure box or in a temperature- controlled container. Specimens that are not frozen are similarly packaged: specimen container, wrapped in absorbent material and placed in individual biohazard bag and secured in transport box of metal or plastic. The specimen may or may not be placed in a temperature-controlled container, depending on ambient temperatures.

Light Considerations in Transporting Specimens and Disposition of Specimens

Most specimens are not sensitive to **light**, but some must be transported in special light-blocking containers or wrapped in aluminum foil during transport: bilirubin, carotene, red cell folate, serum folate, vitamin B2, 6, and 12, and vitamin C. Urine specimens for porphyrins and porphobilinogen must also be protected from light. Light-blocking amber colored collection tubes and urine specimen containers are also available OSHA and state regulations outline the requirements for **disposition** of blood bags and patient samples. Blood disposition must comply with OSHA's Bloodborne Pathogen's Standard (29 CFR 1910.1030), which covers blood (semi-liquid, liquid, dried) in containers, in other waste products, or on items, such as sharps. As a regulated waste, the blood must be placed in a container that is closable, leak-proof, labeled (proper color-coding), and closed before removal to avoid any spillage or loss of contents during transport to disposal site.

Time Considerations When Processing Samples

Specimens should be delivered to the laboratory for processing as quickly as possible and within no more than 45 minutes. Stat tests should be run first. Some tests have **time considerations** that must be followed:

- Blood gases must be processed within 20 minutes.
- Prothrombin time (PT) must be run on unrefrigerated blood sample within 24 hours.
- Partial thromboplastin time (PTT) must be run on room temperature or refrigerated sample within 4 hours.

Additives also affect time considerations:

Additive	Tests	Time from collection
EDTA	Blood smear	Within one hour.
ETDA	CBC	Within 6 hours at room temperature; within 4 hours for micro-collection tubes. However, sample usually stable at room temperature for 24 hours.
EDTA	ESR	With 4 hours at room temperature; within 12 hours if refrigerated.
EDTA	Reticulocyte count	Within 6 hours at room temperature and 72 hours if refrigerated.
Sodium fluoride	Glucose	Within 24 hours at room temperature and 48 hours if refrigerated.

Newborn Screening

While the March of Dimes recommends **newborn screening** for 31 disorders, including hearing deficit, the list of screened diseases varies somewhat, and some states include infectious diseases, such as HIV and toxoplasmosis. All states require testing for PKU, galactosemia, and hypothyroidism, and 44 states and the District of Colombia require at least 29 of the 31 recommended tests. The blood sample should be obtained between 24 and 72 hours after birth because earlier testing may be inaccurate for some disorders, so repeat testing in 2 weeks is required in some states. Tests are carried out through blood spot collection with a heel puncture. The first drop of blood is wiped away, and then a large drop is placed in the center of each circle, being careful to avoid double drops, which may interfere with results, and to fill the circles and penetrate the paper without touching the circles with the child's foot or with the gloved hand. The spot collection papers should be placed horizontally to dry but should not be stacked or hung before or after drying.

PTS

A **pneumatic tube system** (PTS) is an air vacuum system in which carrier tubes are routed through a tubing network to a destination. The PTS can be used to transport laboratory specimens to the laboratory. New systems include barcode tracking, and a computer that maintains records of all transports. The primary advantage of a PTS is that it can markedly decrease turnaround time for processing, especially in large facilities with a centralized laboratory. Carrier tubes are usually made of heavy-duty plastic with foam liners to cushion the sample. There has been some concern about hemolysis of specimens, but studies show the incidence of hemolysis depends on the system, lower than hand-carried specimens with some systems and higher with others, depending on the number of feet traveled per second, the number of direction changes, the total distance, and the gravitational forces. Additionally, some specimens, such as serum samples, are more susceptible to hemolysis or other damage than others. With blood gas analysis, pO2 values may be inaccurate.

Information on Computer-Generated Labels

The label would contain the patient's name, date of birth or age, medical record number, collection time (in military time).

Heparin

The purpose of heparin is to prevent coagulation. The three types of heparin are ammonium, sodium and lithium. Ammonium heparin is used for hematocrit determinations and is found in capillary tubes. Sodium heparin and lithium heparin are used in evacuated tubes. Just be sure that the heparin that is being used is not what is being tested. For example, heparin is used for electrolyte testing, but sodium is a commonly tested electrolyte thus sodium heparin would not be an appropriate heparin to use to test for electrolytes. It is important to mix heparin tubes properly to prevent microclots.

Trace and Ultratrace Elements

Trace elements are metals and may include iron, lead, zinc, mercury, aluminum, and copper. **Ultratrace elements** include boron, nickel, vanadium, arsenic and silicon. Specimens may easily be contaminated so care must be taken to avoid any specimen containers with metal. Special trace-element-free specimen tubes (usually royal blue and containing EDTA, heparin, or no additive) should be used because trace metals may be found in standard glass and plastic tubes and in the stoppers. Because some substances—gadolinium, iodine, and barium contrast—interfere with test results, testing should be delayed for at least 96 hours if patients have received any of these. The specimens must be kept clean and protected from dust. No iodine products should be used for antisepsis, only alcohol. When transferring plasma or serum, it must be poured into aliquots and not transferred by a pipette. Labels are color-coded to indicate the type of additive: lavender indicates EDTA; green, heparin; and red, no additive.

Important Terms

Accession Number: Unique number given for each test request

Aerosol: Substance released in the form of a fine mist

Barcode: Series of black bars and white spaces spaced at intentional, unique distances to represent numbers and letters

Centrifugation: The process of substance separation by spinning

Impermeable: Does not allow the passage of liquids

CPU: Central Processing Unit, the command center of the computer

Cursor: Blinking marker on the computer screen that indicates where information should be inputted

Hardware: The mechanical, magnetic, electronic, and electrical components making up a computer system

Interface: A connection between hardware devices, applications, or different sections of a computer network

Monitor: Aa device similar to a television screen that receives video signals from the computer and displays the information for the user

Support for Clinical Testing

Human Leukocyte Antigens

Human leukocyte antigens (HLA) exist on both tissue cells and white blood cells, and are encoded by genes in the Major Histocompatibility Complex (MHC). This complex is found on the number six chromosome. For transfusions to be successful, human leukocyte antigens must be the same between donor and recipient for all stem cell, tissue, organ, and bone marrow donations. Otherwise, graft versus host disease is likely. Chills and fevers are the most common immune response to the presence of human leukocyte antigens.

Antigen-Antibody Interactions

The interactions between antigens and antibodies may result in the formation of a complex. An antigen will bond to the variable region on the light molecular chain of a corresponding antibody. These interactions may be stronger or weaker depending on the compatibility of the antigens and the antibody. In vitro, the reactions between an antigen and an antibody cause agglutination or hemolysis; in vivo, they may result in an immune response. The following forces conspire to hold together antigen-antibody complexes: hydrophobic bonding, hydrogen bonding, electrostatic charge, and Van der Waal's force.

ABO Blood System

The ABO blood system differentiates based on the amount of A antigens and B antigens on the outside of red blood cells. Individuals who have red blood cells with both A and B antigens on the surface are said to have AB blood. This indicates that such individuals do not have antibodies (IgM) against these antigens in their blood serum. In like fashion, individuals who only have the B antigens on the surface are said to have B blood. Individuals will only have IgM antibodies against the A antigen. Similarly, individuals with type O blood will have red blood cells with neither A nor B antigens on the surface, but blood serum will contain antibodies against both A and B antigens.

The following are the **frequencies of type O, type A, type B, and type AB blood in the** Asian, Black, and Caucasian ethnic groups:

1. Asians: 40% type O; 28% type A; 27% type B; 5% type AB
2. Blacks: 49% type O; 27% type A; 20% type B; 4% type AB
3. Caucasians: 45% type O; 40% type A; 11% type B; 4% type AB

H Antigen

The H antigen is part of the A and B antigens, functioning as an acceptor molecule for sugars. Blood type A is the H antigen with N-acetylgalactosamine affixed. Blood type B is H antigen with D-galactose affixed. Blood type B is also H antigen with no sugar affixed. Only .01% of the world's population has the h antigen rather than the H antigen, known as the Bombay blood group (phenotype hh). These individuals are universal donors because they lack A, B, and H antigens, but can only be transfused with Bombay blood group blood.

Blood Group Systems

Abbreviations and Antibody Classes

The following are abbreviations and antibody classes for blood group systems:

- Kell: abbreviation K; antibody class IgG
- Kidd: Jk; IgG
- Duffy: Fy; IgG

- Lutheran: Lu; IgG and IgM
- Lewis: Le; IgM
- P: P; IgM
- MNS: MNS; IgG and IgM
- Ii: I; IgM

Antigens

The following are antigens related to blood group systems:

- Kell: K (kell), k (Cellano), Kpa, Kpb, Kpc, Jsa, Jsb, K11 (Cote), Wka, and Ku; the most common antigens are K12, K13, K16, K18, K19, K20, and K22
- Duffy: Fya, Fyb, Fy3, Fy4, Fy5, and Fy6
- Kidd: Jka, Jkb, and Jk3
- MNS: M, N, S, s, and U; both of the M and N antigens are associated with glycophorin A; the S, s, and U antigens are associated with glycophorin B

Resistance to Malarial Infection, Hemolytic Disease of Newborn, Mycoplasma Pneumoniae Infection, Chronic Granulomatous Disease, and Paroxysmal Cold Hemoglobinuria

The blood group system or systems related to each are as follows:

- Resistance to malaria: Duffy blood group; phenotype Fy-a-b- is most resistant
- Hemolytic disease of the newborn: related to Rh, ABO, Kell, MNS, and Duffy blood group systems
- Infection with Mycoplasma pneumoniae: related to Ii blood group system
- Chronic granulomatous disease" related to Kell blood group system, especially phenotype K-k-Kp(a-b-)
- Paroxysmal cold hemoglobinuria: related to P blood group system, especially the Donath-Landsteiner antibody

Preparation of Red Blood Cells, Platelets, and Plasma from Whole Blood

Using a centrifuge, lab technicians can separate whole blood into red blood cells, platelets, and plasma. The process is as follows: the bag of whole blood is placed in the centrifuge, immediately separating red blood cells from plasma and platelets. These red blood cells are placed into a separate bag, at which point an additive solution may be mixed in. Plasma and platelets are put into a platelet pack, which is then centrifuged again, separating platelets from plasma. Plasma is put into a fresh frozen plasma bag, while platelets remain in the original container.

Elution

One process that can remove antibodies that are fixed to red blood cells in vivo is called elution. There are three basic kinds of elution:

- Lui freeze-thaw technique: IgM antibodies are removed from the red blood cells of newborn babies
- Digitonin destroys the red blood cells, releasing antibodies
- Intact red blood cell antibody removal (RES): red blood cells are not destroyed, but antibodies are removed using buffers

DAT

The direct antiglobulin test (DAT) detects either IgG antibodies in their blood sample or complement proteins affixed to red blood cells. The test is performed as follows: red blood cells are washed three times with a saline solution, after which antihuman globulin is added. Agglutination at this point indicates the presence of either complement proteins or IgG antibodies. A DAT is often performed in cases of hemolytic disease of the newborn, autoimmune hemolytic anemia, or transfusion reaction.

IAT

The indirect antiglobulin test (IAT) measures the sensitization of red blood cells in vitro. The test is performed as follows: patient's blood serum is mixed with red blood cells and incubated at body temperature. Once the IgG antibodies in the serum have had a chance to attach to the red blood cells, the mixture is washed and antihuman globulin is added. Any agglutination indicates IgG antibodies. A false negative may occur when the washing is not done properly or when antihuman globulin is not added to the solution. A false positive may occur when red blood cells are agglutinated before being washed.

Donath-Landsteiner Test

The Donath-Landsteiner test indicates whether paroxysmal cold hemoglobinuria is present. When this condition is present, individuals will contain hemoglobin cold temperatures. The roots of this disorder are in the anti-P antibody of the P blood group system. This antibody connects to the surfaces of red blood cells in temperatures below 37°C and at warmer temperatures causes hemolysis. The Donath-Lansteiner test is performed as follows: a test tube of serum and red blood cells is placed at 4°C, while a control to his place at 37°C. The test tube of serum and blood is gradually warmed to 37°C, at which point the tubes are centrifuged. If after centrifuging neither displays an indication of hemolysis, the test is negative. When the tube containing serum and red blood cells shows evidence of hemolysis, but the control tube does not, the test is positive. If both tubes show evidence of hemolysis, the test is rendered invalid.

Blood Labeling Requirements

The FDA requires that all blood products and materials used for transfusion be labeled with machine-readable **labeling language** to decrease incidence of errors related to the wrong patient or wrong product. The label must contain at least the unique facility ID, the donor's lot number, the product code, and the blood type of the donor. The two labeling languages in use include:

- Codabar: Labeling that includes an identifying barcode, a description of the contents (such as "RED BLOOD CELLS"), the volume, additives, storage requirements, and test results of FDA required tests (such as HIV and HBV.
- ISB-128: The international standard for identification and labeling as well as transfer of information about body products, including blood. ISB-128 provides a standard terminology, reference tables to apply the appropriate codes, data structures, delivery mechanisms, and standard layout for labels.

Transfusion Record Documentation and Emergent and Routine Transfusion Administration Protocol

Transfusion record documentation must be maintained for at least 5 years and those required for tracing a blood product from donor to disposition maintained for at least 10 years following administration or 5 years after expiration date. Computerized records must be secure and software validated. Records must include all those associated with the donor, recipient, and blood product, including testing (all steps and results), storage, and disposition. The records must be easily accessible and allow for tracing of blood products. Donor records must be maintained and should include information about storage temperatures and visual blood inspections, and preparation of components. Recipient records should include blood type and information regarding antibodies history of transfusions, and adverse transfusion reactions. Records should also be maintained regarding therapeutic phlebotomy, policies and procedures, cytapheresis procedures, antibody identification, quality control, and shipping.

Maintaining Proper Records of All Quality Control and Blood Bank Procedures

Proper **record keeping and documentation** for quality control and blood bank procedures are maintained at 4 different levels:

1. Blood bank polices: A statement of intent that should include the principles that will be utilized to guide decision-making and procedures and may outline the roles and responsibility of employees as well as financial basis for maintaining the program. An example: Employee practices that ensure blood safety.
2. Blood bank processes: These should outline the way things happen, including the chain of command and basic methods of dealing with various functions of the blood bank, such as collecting, storing, and distributing blood products.
3. Blood bank procedures: These are step-by-step explanations of how each blood bank procedure, such as collecting a blood sample or applying a label to a blood product, is carried out, including the equipment and supplies needed.
4. Supporting documentation/Forms: These should include all forms of documentation that are required and samples to show the correct manner of completing and filling out forms required forms.

Storage and Transportation of Blood and Blood Products for Transfusion

The FDA and AAB have established temperature standards for storage and transportation of blood and blood products:

Product	Storage	Transportation
Whole blood, red blood cells (including irradiated, deglycerolized, leukocyte reduced, washed, apheresis), and plasma (including any form after thawing and liquid).	1° to 6°C	1° to 10°C
Platelets (any form), apheresis granulocytes (including irradiated), anti-hemophilic factor (including cryoprecipitated, thawed cryoprecipitated, and plasma thawed cryoprecipitated).	20° to 24°C with continuous agitation	20° to 24°C
Antihemophilic factor (including plasma cryoprecipitated, pooled cryoprecipitated before freezing), plasma (including frozen within 24 hours of phlebotomy and cryoprecipitate reduced).	≤-18°C	Frozen
Fresh frozen plasma	≤-18°C or ≤-65°C	≤-18°C or ≤-65°C

Visible Inspection of Units of Blood/Components

Contamination	Cryoprecipitate	Plasma	Platelets	RBCs
Bacteria	Bubbles, clot, fibrin strains, >opaque	Bubbles, clot, fibrin strains, >opaque	Bubbles, clot, fibrin strains, >opaque, grey appearance	Dk. Purple -> black
Bile	Bright yellow -> brown	Bright yellow -> brown	Bright yellow -> brown	----
Color abnormality	Any abnormal color	Any abnormal color	Any abnormal color	Super natant grey/ brown

VISIBLE INSPECTION OF UNITS OF BLOOD/COMPONENTS

Contamination	Cryo precipitate	Plasma	Platelets	RBCs
Hemolysis	Pink -> red	Pink -> red	----	Bright red
Lipids	White appearance, > opaque	White appearance, > opaque	White appearance, >opaque	Lighter red, >opaque
Particulates	Clots, aggregates of cellular material	t, fibrin strands, white materials	Clot, fibrin strands, white materials	Clots, white materials
RBC contamination	Lt pink -> red	Lt pink -> red	Lt. pink	----

BLOOD BANK REGULATIONS

OSHA and state regulations outline the requirements for **disposition of blood bags and patient samples**. Blood disposition must comply with OSHA's Bloodborne Pathogen's Standard (29 CFR 1910.1030), which covers blood (semi-liquid, liquid, dried) in containers, in other waste products, or on items, such as sharps. As a regulated waste, the blood must be placed in a container that is closable, leak-proof, labeled (proper color-coding), and closed before removal to avoid any spillage or loss of contents during transport to disposal site. **Temperatures:** Blood bank refrigerators are maintained between 2° and 4°C with audible and visible alarm if the temperature falls to 6°C. Freezers are maintained at -20°C, with alerts when the temperature falls to -19°C. Incubators usually provide for a range of temperatures (5° to 70°C) with much incubation done at 37°C. The alarm system for refrigerators, freezers, and incubators should be battery powered so it still functions if the electrical supply is cut.

QUALITY CONTROL FOR ALL REAGENTS

Reagent solutions are used for most diagnostic tests, and results are often dependent on using the correct reagent (stock, working, or standard) at the correct concentration. Quality control procedures include ensuring:

- Accurate weighing and measuring when preparing reagent solutions.
- Carefully following of directions and/or using reagent kits when preparing reagent solutions.
- Choosing the correct reagent.
- Following recommended procedures when disposing of reagents.
- Using proper PPE when working with reagents.
- Neutralizing spilled acids/corrosive chemicals with sodium carbonate or sodium bicarbonate and alkali with dry sand.
- Labeling strong acids and alkali (corrosive compounds) and storing near the floor.
- Properly storing all reagents (acid in glass, flammable reagents in metal or glass, sodium/potassium hydroxide in plastic, hygroscopic chemicals in desiccator or air-tight container, photosensitive chemicals in dark, glass stoppered bottle).
- Monitoring volumes/concentration of chemicals that are explosive when dehydrated.
- Diluting stock only as needed.
- Labeling reagent solutions with date and other information according to directions.
- Labeling all poisonous, flammable, and otherwise hazardous materials.

OPTIMUM STORAGE TEMPERATURES AND EXPIRATION DATES

The optimum storage temperatures and corresponding expiration dates for frozen red blood cells, platelets, cryoprecipitate, pooled platelets, and thawed red blood cells are as follows:

- Frozen red blood cells: -65°C or less; 10 years from collection date
- Platelets: between 20 and 24°C; five days from collection date
- Cryoprecipitate: -18°C or less; one year after collection date

- Pooled platelets: between 20 and 24°C; four hours after pooling
- Thawed red blood cells: between one and 6°C; 24 hours after thawing

Optimum Storage Temperature and Expiration Dates for Red Blood Cells

Any red blood cells that have not been frozen should be stored at temperatures between one and 6 degrees Celsius. If CPD (citrate-phosphate-dextrose) or CP2D (citrate-phosphate-2-dextrose) is the anticoagulant, the expiration date for the red blood cells is three weeks after collection. However, if the anticoagulant is CPDA-1 (citrate-phosphate-dextrose-adenine-one), red blood cells can last five weeks. If the anticoagulants AS-1, AS-2, or AS-3 were used, the red blood cells will last six weeks after collection.

Bacterial Contamination of Blood Products

Occasionally, blood products in storage will suffer a bacterial contamination. The most common type of bacterial contaminant is *Yersinia enterocolitica*. Bacteria of this kind will grow while the product is being stored. Individuals who receive blood products that have been contaminated are likely to manifest symptoms similar to those of an adverse transfusion reaction: fever and chills, e.g. Clots, discoloration, or hemolysis in the blood unit indicates possible contamination.

Transportation Guidelines for Blood Products

Platelets should be transported at room temperature, and they should not be jostled. Red blood cells must be transported at a temperature between one and 10°C; it is standard to place red blood cells in a Styrofoam box inside a cardboard box and on ice. Frozen blood components must be shipped on dry ice and wrapped well.

Therapeutic Phlebotomy

Therapeutic phlebotomy, a blood draw to treat disease, is commonly done to reduce concentration or numbers of red blood cells, ferritin (iron), or porphyrins in the blood for patients with:

- Polycythemia: Increased hemoglobin and hematocrit because of increased red blood cell count that makes blood more viscous.
- Hemochromatosis: Abnormal accumulation of iron in the body, leading to organ damage.
- Porphyrias: Group of disorders in which porphyrins (which are necessary for hemoglobin to function properly) build up in the body.

Blood, usually in about 500 mL units, is withdrawn in a similar manner to blood donations, but most blood is discarded although the FDA allows blood obtained through therapeutic phlebotomy for hemochromatosis to be donated. Patients will have therapeutic phlebotomy on a schedule ordered by the physician, usually to achieve a target hemoglobin. Some patients require blood draws every few days and others once monthly or less frequently.

Hemostasis

Hemostasis is the cessation of bleeding. There are four main steps involved in hemostasis: 1. A damaged blood vessel narrows (vasoconstriction) and the reduced diameter helps slow down any bleeding. 2. Platelets that are present in the blood attach themselves to the collagen in the walls of the blood vessel to create a hemostatic plug within seconds. This process is sometimes referred to as primary hemostasis. After the formation of a hemostatic plug, secondary hemostasis occurs. The clotting factors help fibrin form from fibrinogen. The fibrin then aids in the formation of blood clot at the wound site. Secondary hemostasis takes a few minutes. 3. The newly-formed blood clot helps the wound site create new smooth muscle cells to repair the wound. The clot can then be lyzed (destroyed) when it is not needed any longer.

Platelets

A platelet is a cell fragment is derived from a megakaryocyte. Platelets form in bone marrow, are stored in the spleen, and then move to blood plasma to assist with blood clotting after an injury. Platelets are small, colorless, and irregularly shaped. They have no hemoglobin, no nucleus, and no DNA. Platelets also transport and store several chemicals. A normal platelet count for a healthy adult is between 150,000 and 400,000 per microliter of blood. Platelets are also called thrombocytes.

Fibrin, Heparin, and Plasmin

Fibrin is a protein that aids in blood clotting. Along with platelets, fibrin helps form blood clots. Fibrin is made from the glycoprotein fibrinogen, in the liver. Heparin is a polysaccharide anticoagulant that helps prevent blood clotting. Heparin is concentrated in the vessels surrounding the liver and the lungs. It can also be found in the spleen and various other muscles. Heparin is also a drug that can be given to patients that need to take advantage of its anticoagulant properties, such as in the case of a pulmonary embolism. Plasmin is an enzyme that helps dissolve (lyze) fibrin that is present in blood clots. Lyzing a clot turns coagulated blood into liquid blood again. Plasmin is derived from plasminogen in the blood plasma.

Adjusting Anticoagulant-to-Blood Ratio When Indicated

Anticoagulant-blood ratio adjustment: If a patient's hematocrit is higher than 55%, it is more viscous than normal and contains a lower percentage of plasma. Because of this, for samples collected in a tube with anticoagulant, such as sodium citrate, centrifugation will result in plasma with an increased level of anticoagulant. This, in turn, can affect the test results for all tests run on the sample, so a second sample with anticoagulant corrected should be obtained. For example, a formula is applied to determine the amount of sodium citrate to remove from a tube. For calculation, a 5-mL tube contains 4.5 mL of blood; a 3-mL tube, 2.7 mL; and a 2 mL, 1.8 mL. The volume of sodium citrate for 5-mL tube is 0.5 mL, for the 3-mL tube is 0.3 mL, and for the 2-mL tube is 0.2 mL:

- Sodium citrate volume = $(1.85 \times 10)^{-3} \times (100 - \text{hematocrit}) \times \text{volume of blood}$

Once the volume needed is determined, then the excess anticoagulant is removed from the tube before the blood draw. Correction charts are also available for the various tube sizes. For 5 mL (4.5 mL) tube:

Hematocrit	Sodium citrate volume
57	0.36 mL
63	0.31 mL

Platelet Aggregometer

The platelet aggregometer measures platelet aggregation, when platelets attach to each other to form a clot. Add a coagulation agent, such as ADP, epinephrine, or collagen, to a sample of plasma that showed a high concentration of platelets in the Coulter Counter during the automated CBC. Place the mixture into the aggregometer. The plasma is initially optically dense. As the platelets start to aggregate, the plasma becomes clearer until only serum and the clot remain. In other words, the plasma, with increasing aggregation of platelets, gains the ability to transmit light.

Molecular Testing and Molecular Assays in Coagulation

Molecular testing and molecular assays are used in coagulation studies because they have increased specificity as well as increased sensitivity, and testing can be carried out while the patient is receiving anticoagulant medications. Molecular testing is especially useful for inherited diseases because many coagulation disorders (factor V Leiden mutation, hyperhomocysteinemia, and prothrombin 20210 G>A mutation) and bleeding disorders (hemophilia A and B, von Willebrand disease) involve molecular defects. However, in some cases molecular testing is not practical because of numerous possible mutations, such as with antithrombin testing and protein C and S deficiencies. Numerous different types of procedure are utilized, but one of the most common is the PCR-based assay, especially for inherited clotting disorders, with restriction fragment length polymorphism analysis or other methods. A number of direct hybridization methods, such as the Invader assay, are also available.

Mixing Studies and Factor Testing

Mixing studies are used to determine if abnormal test results for the PT and/or aPTT are because of coagulation deficiency or because of factor inhibitors. Because normal results still occur when PT and aPTT levels are at 50%, the test involves mixing equal amounts of the patient's plasma with a sample of plasma in which the coagulation factors are normal (leading to a 50% level). If the abnormal findings resulted from deficiency, the PT and aPTT results will be within normal range, but if the abnormal findings resulted from inhibitors, then the clotting times will be prolonged.

Factor testing is usually done when the PT and aPTT are abnormally prolonged (or in some cases for thrombosis) to determine the presence and type of clotting abnormality. Factor levels vary, so factor testing generally reports factors as a percentage of normal (which is 100%). Low percentages indicate hypocoagulopathy and percentages above 100% indicate hypercoagulopathy.

Coagulation Procedures

Fibrinogen (factor I)	100-400 mg/dL	Collect 1 mL blood in sodium citrate blue-capped tube (completely filled) for photo-optical clot detection.
		Synthesized in liver, converts to fibrin, which combines with platelets in coagulation sequence. Increased: acute MI, cancer, eclampsia, multiple myeloma, Hodgkin's disease, nephrotic syndrome, tissue trauma. Decreased: DIC, liver disease, congenital fibrinogen abnormality.
Fibrin degradation product (AKA fibrin split products [FSPs])	<5 mcg/mL FEU*	Collect 1 mL blood in sodium citrate blue-capped tube (completely filled) for latex agglutination test. Transport frozen. FSPs occur as clots form and more breakdown of fibrinogen and fibrin occurs, interfering with blood coagulation by coating platelets and disrupting thrombin, and attaching to fibrinogen so stable clots can't form. Increased: DIC, liver disease, MI, hemorrhage, pulmonary embolism, renal disease, obstetric complications, kidney transplant rejection.
Heparin assay (AKA antithrombin III)	1-3 mos: 48-108%.	Collect 1 mL blood in sodium citrate blue-capped tube (completely filled) for chromogenic immunoturbidimetry. Utilized to diagnose heparin resistance in patients receiving heparin therapy and to diagnose hypercoagulable conditions. Increased: Acute hepatitis, kidney transplantation, vit. K deficiency. Decreased: DIC, liver transplantation, nephrotic syndrome, pulmonary embolism, venous thrombosis, liver failure, cirrhosis, carcinoma.
	1-5 yrs.: 82-139%.	
	6-17 yrs.: 90-131%.	
	>18 yrs.: 80-120%.	

Platelet aggregation	Results vary according to laboratory	Collect 4-5 mL sample in sodium citrate tubes for analysis with light transmission aggregometer. Must be processed within 60 minutes of collection. Test measures the ability of platelets to aggregate and form clots in response to various activators. Decreased: Myeloproliferative disorders, autoimmune disorders, uremia, clotting disorders, and adverse effects of medications. Drugs that affect clotting should be avoided before test for up to two weeks (on advice of physician).

FEU = fibrinogen equivalent units

Disposal of Reagents

Laboratories use many different **reagent solutions**, which comprise a solid (solute) dissolved in a liquid (solvent). The three most common types of reagents include:

- Stock: Concentrate that is diluted to prepare a working solution.
- Working: Diluted solution ready for use.
- Standard: Reference solution used to identify the concentration of other solutions.

Reagents may be classified as solid wastes (which can include liquids) or hazardous wastes. Some reagents, such as those containing sodium azide, must be disposed of as hazardous waste in hazardous waste drums and sent to hazardous waste facilities for incineration (most hazardous wastes cannot go into landfills), but some others, such as ethanol diluted to less than 24%, may be discharged into the sewer. Some, such as DAB, may be detoxified before sewer disposal. Manufacturer's directions for disposal must be followed for each reagent.

Loading an Analyzer

Automated analyzers (hematology) carry out the CBC and differentials and chemical analyzers carry out numerous chemical tests. Some analyzers are small and process one blood sample at a time. Others are able to process hundreds of samples (usually serum or plasma), which are placed in tubes or special cups, labeled, and loaded into the analyzer in racks or carousels. Some machines now allow capped specimens to be processed, reducing the risk of exposure. Procedures vary according to the type of analyzer and the manufacturer, but all analyzers require some types of reagents to carry out tests. The expiration dates and volumes of the various reagents should be checked as part of daily maintenance and containers replaced and/or refilled as necessary. With some equipment, checking is done automatically. As part of daily maintenance, controls and calibrators with known values are loaded into the analyzers and tested to determine if the results are accurate.

Technical and Analytical Error Recognition Related to Analyzers and Reporting

While most **errors** related to analysis of laboratory specimens are preanalytical (related to collection, transport, storage, or preparation), some errors result from problems with the analyzers themselves. Errors may result from:

- Equipment malfunction: This may result from power failure, computer error, damaged equipment or machine part. Most newer equipment has alarms to alert to processing problems, but older or less costly equipment many not. The equipment may not be calibrated correctly, so carrying out calibration and quality control testing is essential.

- Specimen problems: Hemolysis, coagulation, or various other problems may render the specimen inadequate for testing.
- Reagents: The incorrect reagent may have been loaded into the analyzer or the reagent may be expired, defective, or contaminated.

Any errors found must be reported to a supervisor immediately and processing of samples stopped until troubleshooting is carried out to determine the cause of the errors. Depending on when the error was noted, some tests may need to be rerun.

Photomultiplier Tube

A photomultiplier tube converts light to electrical currents. This conversion to electricity is extremely rapid. In addition, the tube amplifies the signal that is received. This amplification can be very high, up to one million times amplification. To accomplish this conversion, as well as the amplification, a very high internal voltage must be present. The voltage can be as high as 1500 volts.

Turbidimetry

Turbidimetry is a measurement of the quantity of light that is blocked by particles in a solution as the light passes through that solution (turbidity). There are several problems inherent in this technique, however. In order to compare the turbidity of a sample with a standard, the quantity and number of particles present in both the sample and the standard must be similar or comparable. Any great variation in particle size between the particles present in the sample and the particles present in the standard can be problematic. Also, any settling and/or aggregation of particles present can be a problem in obtaining accurate results. Consistent timing in the preparation of the samples is therefore extremely necessary to avoid this issue.

Flame Emission Photometry

Flame emission photometry is based on the fact that excited electrons release extra energy (light) when the electrons drop down to their stable ground state. For example, when a metallic element (such as Na+, K+, or Li+) absorbs energy (in the form of heat), the orbital electrons of that element move to a higher, unstable energy level from the stable ground state. These electrons are now called "excited electrons". Since the excited electrons are at an unstable energy level, the drop back down to their ground state, to achieve a stable energy. As the electrons do this, they release their extra energy in the form of light. The light is released at a specific wavelength, depending on the element in question. Each element has a unique wavelength associated with it. Furthermore, the quantity of light that is released is directly related to the amount of the particular element present.

Mass Spectrometry

Mass spectrometry is a technique used in the identification of compounds. This identification is accomplished using a mass spectrometer. A mass spectrometer determines the mass (molecular weight) to charge ratio of ions in the sample being tested. A mass spectrum can then be created which shows the masses of the components (ions) present in the sample. In the creation of the mass spectrum, magnetic and/or electric fields are used to sort the ions. Mass spectrometry is useful in identifying drugs in the lab, and it can be used in conjunction with a variety of other laboratory techniques, such as gas-liquid chromatography.

Used in Conjunction with Gas-Liquid Chromatography in the Lab

Mass spectrometry can be used in conjunction with gas-liquid chromatography in the lab to aid the technician in the proper identification of a sample. Certain compounds, albeit different compounds from each other, can have similar retention times. Gas-liquid chromatography uses retention times to identify compounds. Therefore, if several compounds have similar retention times, the compound in question can be misidentified using gas-liquid chromatography alone. However, if the peak resulting from a gas-liquid chromatography analysis is taken to a mass spectrometer for analysis on the basis of mass, the particular compound in question can be correctly identified.

Electrolytic Cells

An electrolytic cell consists of three main parts: an anode, a cathode, and an electrolytic solution. When electricity is applied to an electrolytic cell, an internal chemical reaction in the cell between the ions present in the electrolytic solution and the anode or cathode occurs. The electrolytic solution is composed of water and other solvents, for the purpose of dissolving ions in the solution. The anode is a positively charged electrode, and negatively charged ions (anions) flow toward the anode. These ions are oxidized, or lose electrons, at the anode. The cathode is a negatively charged electrode, and positively charged ions (cations) flow toward the cathode. These ions are reduced, or gain electrons, at the cathode.

Operation of Nephelometer

Nephelometers measure concentration of particulates in gas or liquid. In medicine, nephelometry is used to measure the levels of blood protein (immunoglobulins) when assessing immune function and can detect antigens or antibodies with a light beam (usually laser) according to light-scattering properties. Nephelometers are commonly used outside of medicine to measure air quality, including visibility. Many different types of nephelometers are available and may operate slightly differently:

- Gather supplies.
- Calibrate with standard at 1:80, 1:160 and continue doubling to 1:2560 according to manufacturer's guidelines
- Load specimen into serum racks and reagent into reagent racks.
- Adjust equipment to proper setting for test.
- Run sample.
- Remove sample and reagent.
- Shut down equipment.

Operation of Osmometers

Osmometers measure the osmotic pressure, vapor pressure, and osmotic strength of solutions. Many different types of osmometers (vapor pressure depression, freezing point depression, membrane) are available and may operate slightly differently. Osmometers are commonly used to assess the concentrations (osmolality) of salts and sugars present in blood of urine:

- Gather reagents and equipment.
- Follow manufacturers guidelines for calibration (often done automatically) with sampler, which usually requires analysis of 2 calibration standards. Calibration standards include 1500 mOsm/kg and 850 mOsm/kg. Complete calibration and utilize chamber cleaner if needed.
- Draw sample into sampler and insert sampler into testing chamber.
- Press start button and wait for results, remove sampler and clean chamber.

Immunoassay and Electrophoresis

Immunoassays utilize antigens or antibodies to test for the presence of disease. For example, an antigen may be used to test for the presence of antibodies in a blood sample. If present, the antibody will bind to the antigen. Immunoassays that identify target antibodies include tests for rheumatoid factor, West Nile virus, and hepatitis B. Immunoassays that target antigens include tests for levels of drugs (digoxin), levels of hormones (testosterone, insulin), and markers of cancer (PSA).

Electrophoresis involves application of an electrical field to macromolecules (RNA, DNA, and proteins) suspended in liquid on various media in order to separate them by size. A charge (negative or positive) causes macromolecules to move toward the opposite charge. Electrophoresis may be used to study DNA or RNA and may help to diagnosis disorders that involve abnormal proteins, such as some types of cancer, renal disease, and multiple sclerosis. Electrophoresis is also used to test vaccines and antibiotics.

Preventive Maintenance on Laboratory Equipment

A medical technologist should perform preventive maintenance for several reasons. For one, as equipment is used, parts can tend to wear out or even break. For best equipment performance, these worn out parts should be replaced regularly. Calibration and other adjustments should also be made on a regular basis so equipment can give the most accurate results in laboratory tests. Preventive maintenance is also important for keeping instruments and equipment clean. Following all preventive maintenance schedules will keep laboratory equipment running smoothly, and will also keep all equipment functioning for as long as possible.

Discrete Analyzers and Continuous Flow Analyzers

A discrete analyzer is an analyzer in which all specimens and samples are analyzed separately. The specimens each have their own individual vessels for analysis. An example of a discrete analyzer is the Automated Clinical Analyzer (ACA). A continuous flow analyzer is an analyzer in which all samples flow through the same tubing during analysis. In addition, the samples flow in a continuous stream. To separate the samples analyzed in a continuous flow analyzer, air bubbles are used. An example of a continuous flow analyzer is the Sequential Multiple Analyzer Computer (SMAC).

Chemistry Analyzer Maintenance

Maintenance of the chemistry analyzer will vary depending on the types and size, with some requiring much more hands-on maintenance and manual calibration than others. General maintenance requirements include:

- Check location of installation (electrical, infrastructure), including voltage, outlet polarity, and space for ventilation and cables.
- Assess security and cleanliness.
- Assess exposure to thermal radiation, vibration, excess humidity, excess temperature, dust, smoke, and corrosive materials/emissions.
- Check any lights and on/off or command buttons to make sure they are functioning.
- Check printer.
- Clean any spills, breakage.
- Ensure equipment is covered when not in use.
- Ensure proper calibration is carried out.
- If the equipment has fuses, replace as needed.
- For small equipment, ensure it is disconnected from power after use.
- Carry out routine scheduled maintenance, daily, weekly, monthly, every 6 months, and annually according to manufacturer's guidelines.

Shift and Trend on Quality Control Charts

A shift is said to have occurred when the control values on a quality control chart appear to have changed suddenly. Also, if the control values on the quality control chart are consistently being found to be higher or lower than the mean value (within two standard deviations) on several days in a row in the laboratory, a shift is said to have occurred. A trend on a quality control chart, on the other hand, is a gradual, fairly slow change in control values over a time period of several days. This is in contrast to the abrupt change in control values that characterizes a shift.

Causes of Upward Shift, Downward Shift, and Trend on Quality Control Charts

An upward shift on a quality control chart may be caused by the change to a new standard that has a lower concentration than what is required for the particular test being performed. A downward shift, on the other hand, can be caused by the change to a new standard that has a higher concentration than what is required for the particular test being performed. A trend on a quality control chart is most often caused by a slow deterioration or breaking down of an instrument, piece of equipment, or a reagent. A trend can be either downwards or upwards.

Quality Assurance

Quality assurance involves the monitoring and checking of all aspects of the medical laboratory. A laboratory quality assurance program involves several aspects. For one, all instruments and equipment should be checked on a regular basis. Making sure that all parts are in working order and are performing as expected is very important. This is also a part of the preventive maintenance program. Specimen collection and labeling should also be monitored. Correct collection and labeling of specimens is an important step in obtaining accurate laboratory results. All laboratory supplies, equipment, and even water should also be reviewed. All supplies should meet all necessary specifications, and should be in found in working order. Finally, the precision and accuracy of all laboratory results and analyses should be a priority. Quality control charts, appropriate controls and standards should all be used. A laboratory's participation in an external survey program, such as one from the American Society of Clinical Pathologists (ASCP) will also help a laboratory maintain its quality assurance.

Procedures When a Group of Test Results Appear to Be Out of Control

When a group of test results appears to be out of control, the troubleshooting procedures for the test method in question must be followed. As part of the laboratory's quality control program, these troubleshooting procedures should already be written and developed for use in cases such as these. The instructions will likely tell the technician to check any and all calculations that have been made, to make a visual inspection of all reagents that have been used, and to inspect all instruments and equipment that have been used as well. After these steps have been accomplished to satisfaction, the technician may be instructed to rerun a set of tests with a new sample of the control. In discovering a group of out of control test results, the technician is not to inform the doctor ordering the tests of the out of control results. Also, the technician should be sure to not change batches of standards or reagents used, as this will affect the results obtained.

Laboratory Standards and Integrity Assessment

Laboratory standards are established by a number of agencies, including OSHA, which establishes safety standards; the EPA, which established good laboratory practices; CLSI, which provides global laboratory standards; and ISO-9000, which establishes standards for quality management. Laboratory standards are norms or requirements stablished for the profession. **Integrity assessment** is carried out to determine if a laboratory is meeting standards or has engaged in fraud or misconduct (as opposed to accidents or errors), such as through:

- Failure to properly carry out procedures.
- Falsification of records or measurements, incomplete documentation, manipulation of data.
- Violation of standards or rules of conduct, violations of codes of ethics.
- Misrepresentation of quality assurance results.
- Failure to adequately calibrate equipment.
- Failure to retain samples for required time.
- Improper storage of reagents, samples, and supplies.
- Failure to follow standard operating procedures.
- Alterations of log book.
- Employment of personnel without appropriate license or certification.

Integrity assessment may include reviewing data, comparing manual logs with computer logs, conducting an audit trail, carrying out unannounced audits, encouraging and supporting whistleblowers.

Formation of Creatinine

Creatinine is formed from free creatine. Creatine is formed from various amino acids, including glycine, arginine, and methionine. Guanidinoacetate is formed from a reaction between glycine and arginine in various body tissues, including the liver, pancreas, and the kidneys. The guanidinoacetate is moved to the liver via the blood, where it reacts with *S*-adenosylmethionine to form creatine. The creatine is then transported to various muscle tissues via the blood system. This creatine is found in the form of phosphocreatine in the muscle tissues. Phosphocreatine is a high energy compound and helps form ATP by supplying phosphate for the formation. ATP is very important for muscle metabolism. When the ATP is formed, there is also a release of free creatine. The free creatine then transforms in the creatinine through an irreversible and spontaneous reaction. Creatinine is excreted as a waste product in human urine, and serves no functional purpose in the human body.

Performing Common Renal Function Tests

Non-protein nitrogens: Creatinine, BUN, uric acid, and ammonia	Collect 1 mL serum in red or tiger-capped tube or 1 mL plasma in heparinized green-capped tube. Uric acid—If patient is receiving rasburicase, the specimen must be obtained in a pre-chilled heparinized tube and transported in ice slurry. Ammonia—1 mL plasma in EDTA lavender capped tube or heparinized green-capped tube (tightly capped) and transported in ice slurry. Method of testing for all: Spectrophotometry.
Creatinine clearance Reference value: 70-130 mL/min/1.73^2	Patients should avoid strenuous exercise for 48 hours before beginning test and meat/other protein restricted to ≤8 ounces for 24 hours before beginning test. Collection begins after disposing of first morning urine. A blood specimen is usually also taken for a serum creatinine. Urine is collected for a 24-hour period and stored at room temperature. Urine is mixed and measured and a specimen transferred for creatinine testing. Data are entered into computer (age, height, weight, ethnicity if appropriate).
Estimated glomerular filtration rate (eGFR) Reference value: >90 mL/min/1.73^2 <60 ml/min/1.73^2 indicates kidney disease	• The eGFR is not directly measured but is estimated based on serum creatinine levels. • Various formulas are used to estimate the GFR: • General (adults): (Urine Creatinine / Serum Creatinine) × Urine Volume (mL) / [time (hr) X 60] = eGFR. • Schwartz (children): (k) × height in cm/ serum creatinine = GFR (mL/min/1.73m^2). • k = Constant (muscle mass) • k = 0.33 in premature infants • k = 0.45 in term infants to 1 year old • k = 0.55 in children to 13 years and adolescent females • k = 0.65 in adolescent males • Modified MDRD formula for 18-70 years: GFR (mL/min/1.73 m^2) = 175 x (Scr)$^{-1.154}$ x (Age)$^{-0.203}$ x (0.742 if female) x (1.212 if African American) (conventional units).

Renal Function Tests

Specific gravity	1.015-1.025. Determines kidney's ability to concentrate urinary solutes. Increased: dehydration, diabetes, fever, CHF, and adrenal insufficiency. Decreased: diuresis, hypervolemia, hypothermia, and renal disease (impaired concentrating ability)
Osmolality (urine)	350-900 mOsm/kg/24 hours. Shows early defects if kidney's ability to concentrate urine is impaired. Increased: CHF, dehydration, SIADH, and azotemia. Decreased: diabetes insipidus, hypernatremia, hypokalemia, and primary polydipsia.
Osmolality (serum)	275-295 mOsm/kg. Increased: Azotemia, dehydration, diabetes insipidus, diabetic ketoacidosis, hypercalcemia, and hypernatremia. Decreased: adrenocorticoid insufficiency, hyponatremia, SIADH, and water intoxication.
Creatinine clearance (24-hour)	Male 85-125 mL/min/1.73 m^2, Female 75-115 mL/min/1.73 m^2. Evaluates the amount of blood cleared of creatinine in 1 minute. Approximates the glomerular filtration rate.
Serum creatinine	0.6-1.2 mg/dL. Level should remain stable with normal functioning. Increased: acromegaly, CHF, poliomyelitis, renal disease, shock, and rhabdomyolysis. Decreased: loss of muscle mass, hyperthyroidism, inadequate protein intake, liver disease, muscular dystrophy, and pregnancy.
Urine creatinine	Male 14-26 mg/kg/24 hr, Female 11-20 mg/kg/24 hr. Increased: acromegaly, carnivorous diets, exercise, and gigantism. Decreased: glomerulonephritis, pyelonephritis, leukemia, muscle wasting disorders, PKD, shock, urinary tract obstructions, and vegetarian diets.
Blood urea nitrogen (BUN)	7-8 mg/dL (8-20 mg/dL >60 years of age). Increased: impaired renal function (as urea is end product of protein metabolism), chronic glomerulonephritis, CHF, diabetes, GI bleeding, hypovolemia, ketoacidosis, starvation (muscle wasting), neoplasm, pyelonephritis, shock, nephrotoxic agents, and urinary tract obstruction. Decreased: inadequate protein intake, low protein diet, malabsorption syndromes, pregnancy, and liver disease.
BUN/ creatinine ratio	10:1. Increases with hypovolemia. With intrinsic kidney disease, the ratio is normal, but the BUN and creatinine are increased.
Uric acid	Male 4.4-7.6, Female 2.3-6.6 mg/dL. Increased: renal failure, gout, pernicious anemia, and sickle cell anemia. Decreased: chronic alcoholism, hypertension, and renal disease.

Jaffe Reaction for Creatinine Determination

The Jaffe reaction is the basis for most creatinine determination methods. It is based on the fact that creatinine reacts with an alkaline picrate solution. This reaction produces a bright orange-red compound, indicating the presence of creatinine. There is a major drawback to the Jaffe reaction, however. This drawback is that it has a lack of specificity for creatinine. Several other compounds can react with an alkaline picrate solution, such as glucose and various proteins. Using Lloyd's reagent can help with this drawback however. Lloyd's reagent is an aluminum silicate that can adsorb creatinine. This aids in the separation of creatinine from some of the competing compounds before the development of the orange-red compound.

Mathematical Equation for Creatinine Clearance

Average Sized Adult

The creatinine clearance for an average sized adult, in milliliters per minute (mL/min), can be calculated by the equation U/P x V. In this equation, U represents the creatinine concentration in the urine, in milligrams per deciliter (mg/dL), P represents the creatinine concentration in the plasma, in milligrams per deciliter (mg/dL), and V represents the volume of urine per minute, with the volume expressed in milliliters. Use the conversion factor of 24 hours being equal to 1440 minutes to convert the volume of urine over a 24 hour period to the volume of urine per minute. One thing to keep in mind with calculating the creatinine clearance is that the body surface area and the kidney size of an individual can affect the creatinine clearance. In an average sized individual, these factors are not really taken into account.

Infant

When calculating creatinine clearance for an infant, we need to take into account the body surface area of the infant. Therefore, use the equation U/P x V x 1.73/A to calculate the creatinine clearance of an infant (mL/min/standard surface area). In this equation, U represents the creatinine concentration in the urine in milligrams per deciliter (mg/dL), P represents the creatinine concentration in the plasma in milligrams per deciliter (mg/dL), and V represents the volume of urine per minute with the volume expressed in milliliters. Use the conversion factor of 24 hours being equal to 1440 minutes to convert the volume of urine over a 24-hour period to the volume of urine per minute. 1.73 represents the average body surface area in square meters (m^2) of an average sized adult. A is the body surface area in square meters (m^2) of the individual (the infant) in question.

Ultraviolet Procedure for Quantifying Uric Acid

The ultraviolet procedure for quantifying uric acid is based on the principle that uric acid absorbs ultraviolet light in the region of 290—293 nm. If uricase is added to uric acid, the uricase will destroy the uric acid. This happens because the uricase acts as a catalyst helping to break down the uric acid to carbon dioxide and allantoin. Because of this breakdown and the ability of uric acid to absorb ultraviolet light, differential spectrophotometry can be used to quantify uric acid in a sample. The ultraviolet procedure is accomplished using centrifugal fast-analyzer systems. These systems have the ability to monitor the decreasing absorbance of ultraviolet light as the uric acid is destroyed by uricase. As the uric acid is destroyed, and its concentration in a specimen decreases, the absorbance of ultraviolet light also proportionally decreases.

Physical and Chemical Properties of Urine

Color	Pale yellow/ amber and darkens when urine is concentrated or other substances (such as blood or bile) or present.
Appearance	Clear but may be slightly cloudy.
Odor	Slight. Bacteria may give urine a foul smell, depending upon the organism. Some foods, such as asparagus, change odor.
Specific gravity	1.015 to 1.025. May increase if protein levels increase or if there is fever, vomiting, or dehydration.
pH	Usually ranges between 4.5 and 8, with average of 5 to 6.
Sediment	Red cell casts from acute infections, broad casts from kidney disorders, and white cell casts from pyelonephritis. Leukocytes >10/ml^3 are present with urinary tract infections.
Glucose, ketones, protein, blood, bilirubin, and nitrate	Negative. Urine glucose may increase with infection (with normal blood glucose). Frank blood may be caused by some parasites and diseases but also by drugs, smoking, excessive exercise, and menstrual fluids. Increased red blood cells may result from lower urinary tract infections.
Urobilinogen	0.1-1.0 units. Increased in liver disease.

Benedict's Test

Benedict's test is a laboratory test that is used to determine the presence of reducing substances in a urine sample. Some reducing substances that can be present in urine include glucose (which can be indicative of diabetes), other reducing sugars such as lactose and galactose, creatinine, uric acid, or ascorbic acid. The test can tell a technician or a doctor if reducing substances are present in the urine sample, but the test itself is nonspecific. In other words, the test cannot determine the specific reducing substance present. To perform the test, Benedict's reagent (a solution of copper sulfate, sodium carbonate, and sodium citrate) is added to a urine sample, and the mixture is heated. A red, yellow, or orange precipitate is indicative of the presence of a reducing substance in the urine. The precipitate is formed because the copper sulfate in the Benedict's reagent is reduced by any reducing substance contained in the urine.

Addis Count Procedure

The Addis count is a laboratory technique to calculate the number of formed elements in a urine sample. The formed elements include blood cells (white blood cells and red blood cells) and casts. In this test, a twelve-hour urine specimen is collected. Formalin is used as a preservative for the urine sample. After the twelve-hour period, a specified quantity of the urine specimen is put in a centrifuge. Part of any resuspended urine sediment is then placed into a Neubauer blood-counting chamber. The squares of the blood-counting chamber are then examined. Any formed elements, such as casts, white blood cells, or red blood cells, that are present are counted. The total number of formed elements in the entire urine sample is then calculated. This test can be used on the urine of patients that have kidney disease.

HCG Hemagglutination Inhibition Test

The HCG hemagglutination test is used to determine pregnancy by examining a urine sample. Add a sample of urine to two drops of HCG antiserum. To this, add red blood cells that have been coated in HCG. If HCG is present in the urine sample, the HCG antiserum binds to the HCG present, therefore making it impossible for the HCG antiserum to react with the red blood cells coated in HCG. This leads to the red cells not agglutinating, and a donut shape consisting of red blood cells will form. This donut shape indicates HCG in the urine sample. However, if there is no HCG present in the urine sample, the HCG antiserum will bind with the HCG coated red blood cells. No donut pattern of red blood cells will form. Instead, there will be a diffuse pattern of red blood cells. This diffuse pattern indicates that no HCG is present in the urine sample. The patient is not pregnant, or is pregnant more than six months.

Confirmatory Urine Tests

Clinitest®	Confirms the presence of glucose in the urine. Drop alkaline copper reagent tables in a tube containing 5 drops of urine and 10 drops of distilled water, which will boil. Wait 15 seconds after boiling stops, gently shake tube, and check color against chart. Blue is negative and colors from green to orange indicate the presence of 1/4% (+) to 2% (++++) glucose.
Ictotest®	Confirms the presence of bilirubin in the urine. Place 10 drops of urine on a special absorbant mat, place a reagent table in the middle of the moistened are and then one drop of distilled water on the tablet. After 5 seconds, place another drop of distilled water on the table. Wait 60 seconds and observe the color about and under the tablet. Blue or purple color indicates the presence of bilirubin.
Acetest® (Acetone test)	Confirms the presence of ketones in the urine. Place tablet on clean dry white paper and place 1 drop of urine on top of tablet. Wait 30 seconds and check color against color chart. No change in color is negative and shades of lavender (light, medium, and dark) indicate small, moderate, and large amounts of ketones.
Sulfosalicylic acid (SSA)	Confirms the presence of protein in the urine. If urine is cloudy, centrifuge before test. Fill tube (10 × 75 mm) one-third full of urine and add one-third tube of 3% SSA solution. Cover with paraffin film/cap and mix by inverting. Check results by holding in front of lined/text test strip. If the lines/text are clear, the result is negative, slightly cloudy but lines/text visible, 1+; lines are visible but unable to read text, 2+; no lines/text visible, 3+; totally opaque/gelled, 4+.

Orthostatic Proteinuria

Orthostatic proteinuria (also referred to as postural proteinuria) is a condition that is characterized by an excessive amount of protein (usually albumin) that is excreted into urine as a function of the patient's position. Usually, during the day, when the patient is upright (sitting or standing), there is an increased amount of protein excreted into the urine. At night, however, when the patient is lying down, there is a normal amount of protein excreted into the urine. This condition affects adolescents mostly between the ages of ten and twenty, and up to three to five percent of adolescents are affected with orthostatic proteinuria. Affected people, other than the excessive protein excretion, have no other health problems or issues, and for the most part, appear to be healthy. In the laboratory, the existence of this condition can be determined by comparing urine samples taken during the day, and ones taken at night, or right after a person awakes from sleeping.

Residual Urine

Residual urine is the volume of urine that remains in the bladder after urination. The normal residual volume is less than 50 mL although a residual volume of less than 100 mL may be acceptable in older patients, as the bladder may not contract as efficiently as in younger adults. If the bladder does not empty completely, such as may occur in males with blockage from enlarged prostates, the patient is at increased risk of urinary tract infection and bladder distention. Patients may feel an almost constant need to urinate and may dribble urine. Post-void residual urine volume may be assessed through ultrasound. Residual urine volume may be assessed more accurately through catheterization. **Types of catheters** include:

- Continuous drainage (Foley®) catheters: Catheter inserted into bladder and balloon inflated to hold the catheter in place. Catheter attached to tubing and collection bag.
- Intermittent (straight) catheters: Disposable or reusable catheter inserted into bladder to drain urine and then removed.
- External catheters: Applied like a condom to the penis with tubing and a collection bag attached. Used primarily for males with incontinence, but may be used to obtain a urine specimen although not for residual urine.

Bilirubin

Bilirubin is the breakdown product that is derived from the degradation of the heme in hemoglobin. It is the reddish-yellow pigment of bile, and it can either be described as being conjugated (water-soluble in blood) or unconjugated (bound to albumin). The formation of bilirubin starts with the breakdown of hemoglobin in old (dying) red blood cells. This breakdown is very rapid in certain cells of the bone marrow, spleen, and liver. First, the globin protein is denatured and removed from the hemoglobin in the red blood cells. Then, the tetrapyrrole ring (4 pyrroles in a ring) of the heme is oxidized and opened up. Iron is then added and the green pigment biliverdin is formed. Biliverdin is then reduced by the addition of hydrogen to form bilirubin.

Hemoglobin

Hemoglobin is an iron-containing protein that is used to transport oxygen from the lungs to other body tissues. The iron in the hemoglobin is what gives blood its characteristic red color. Hemoglobin contains 4 iron atoms, 4 heme groups, and 4 globin chains (or protein groups). Hemoglobin contains approximately 94% globin and 6% heme. In addition, hemoglobin is produced in the bone marrow by erythrocytes. The most common form of hemoglobin in an adult is hemoglobin A.

Jaundice

Jaundice is a condition that is characterized by the yellowing of certain parts of the body, such as the skin, the sclera (whites of the eyes) and the mucous membranes. Jaundice is due to an increased amount of bilirubin in the blood plasma. The bilirubin can either be conjugated bilirubin or unconjugated bilirubin (conjugated jaundice or unconjugated jaundice). Jaundice is said to be present when the total bilirubin levels are greater than 2.5 mg/dL. The increased amount of bilirubin in the blood can be due to several things. For one, there could be an obstruction in the bile duct of the liver (obstructive jaundice). There could also be an increase in the breakdown of blood in the body, causing increased bilirubin levels (hemolytic jaundice), or liver cells could be damaged (parenchymal jaundice). Jaundice can also be due to a combination of these factors.

Review Video: Jaundice/Icterus
Visit mometrix.com/academy and enter code: 339680

Common Hepatic Function Tests

Bilirubin	Collect sample in heparinized green-capped tube, 0.6 mL blood, centrifuge to volume of 0.2 mL plasma/serum. Sample must be protected from light and analyzed within 2 hours. Refrigerate for storage. Test in chemical analyzer or photometric assay according to manufacturer's directions.
Albumin	Collect sample in red top with or without clot activator or heparinized green-top tube for test on serum or plasma. Test in chemical analyzer according to manufacturer's directions.
Prothrombin time (PT)	Sample should completely fill blue-capped tube with inversions immediately after drawing. Do not centrifuge or freeze if sample must be transported. Test in coagulometer.
Alkaline phosphatase (ALP)	Patient should fast 8-12 hours before test. Sample collected in gel-barrier tube and centrifuged as soon as possible for complete separation. Test in chemical analyzer.
Aspartate aminotransferase (AST)	Sample collected in gel-barrier tube, centrifuged for complete separation, and stored in refrigerator. Test in chemical analyzer according to manufacturer's directions.
Alanine transferase (ALT)	Same as AST.
Gamma-glutamyl transpeptidase (GGT)	Same as AST. Separate as soon as possible.
Ammonia	Sample collected in 1 mL plasma in EDTA lavender capped tube or heparinized green-capped tube (tightly capped) and transported in ice slurry. Centrifuge within 15 minutes without removing stopper, separate plasma and freeze in plastic vial. Test through micro-diffusion apparatus (indirect), enzymatic method (direct) with glutamate dehydrogenase or ammonium electrode, or ammonia analyzer.
Cholesterol	Patient should fast for 12 hours. Collect sample in red top with or without clot activator or heparinized green-top tube for test on serum or plasma. Store serum in refrigerator. Test in analyzer.

Hepatic Function Test Results

Bilirubin	Determines the ability of the liver to conjugate and excrete bilirubin: direct 0.0-0.3 mg/dL, total 0.0-0.9 mg/dL, and urine 0. Increased: Hemolytic jaundice, hemolytic anemia, liver disease, anorexia nervosa, hypothyroidism, and obstructive jaundice.
Albumin	1. Albumin: 4.0-5.5 g/dL. Primary protein found in the liver. Decreased: Liver disease, malabsorption, malnutrition, chronic diseases, parasitic infections, prolonged immobilization, burns, kidney disease, pre-eclampsia, overhydration, Cushing disease, and enteropathies.

	2. Albumin/globulin (A/G) ratio: 1.5:1 to 2.5:1. Albumin should be greater than globulin. Abnormalities occur with liver disease.
Prothrombin time (PT)	100% or clot detection in 10 to 13 seconds. Increased: Liver disease, coagulation disorders, massive transfusions, celiac disease, salicylate overdose, vitamin K deficiency, and chronic diarrhea. Decreased: Ovarian hyperfunction and ileitis.
Alkaline phosphatase (ALP)	17-142 adults. (Normal values vary with method.) Indicates biliary tract obstruction if no bone disease. Increased: Liver tumor, hepatitis, aplastic anemia, Hodgkin's disease, multiple myeloma, polycythemia vera, leukemias, thrombocytopenia. Decreased: Sickle cell and sideroblastic anemia.
Aspartate aminotransferase (AST)	10-40 units. Increased: Liver cell damage, hepatitis, pancreatitis, shock, cardiac arrhythmias, CHF, muscle disease, MI, CVA, and DTs. Decreased: Hemodialysis, vitamin B-6 deficiency, and uremia.
Alanine transferase (ALT)	5-35 units. Increased: Liver cell damage, pancreatitis, AIDS, burns, muscle injury, muscular dystrophy, myositis, shock, and pre-eclampsia. Decreased: Pyridoxal phosphate deficiency.
Gamma-glutamyl transpeptidase (GGT)	5-55 μ/L females, 5-85 μ/L males. Increased: Alcohol abuse, liver disease, hyperthyroidism, mononucleosis, pancreatitis, and renal transplantation. Decreased: Hypothyroidism.
Lactate dehydrogenase (LDH)	100-200 units. Increased: Alcohol abuse, hepatic carcinoma, hemolytic anemias, leukemias, MI or pulmonary infarction, pancreatitis, shock, viral hepatitis, and renal disease.
Serum ammonia	150-250 mg/dL. Increased: Liver failure, GI hemorrhage, inborn deficiency, and total parenteral nutrition.
Cholesterol	<200 mg/dL. Increased: Bile duct obstruction, diabetes, glomerulonephritis, gout, hypothyroidism, nephrotic syndrome, obesity, pregnancy, syndrome X, and anorexia nervosa. Decreased: Hepatic parenchymal disease, pernicious anemia, hyperthyroidism, COPD, leukemia (CML), thalassemia, sideroblastic anemia, and myeloma.

Test Elevations with Liver Disease or Obstructive and Hemolytic Jaundice

Cirrhosis	Generally, values of hepatic function tests elevated. Creatinine clearance falls with hepatorenal syndrome and serum creatinine increases; ammonia levels increase with hepatic encephalopathy.
Liver failure	Elevation of AST, GGT, ALT, ASP, lactate, ammonia, and bilirubin.
Viral hepatitis	Elevation of bilirubin (serum and urine), ALP may elevate with biliary obstruction/abscess, PT may be prolonged. Serum ammonia may be elevated (with altered mental status). AST, ALT, and GTT may be elevated.
Obstructive jaundice	Serum bilirubin, ALP, and GTT are elevated. AST is usually not elevated unless complications occur. PT may be prolonged. Urine bilirubin is usually not present.
Hemolytic jaundice	Elevation of unconjugated bilirubin and LDH.

Laboratory Methods to Determine Serum Bilirubin Concentration

The following are laboratory methods used to determine serum bilirubin concentration:

- Bilirubin Oxidase: In this method, bilirubin oxidase, an enzyme, serves as a catalyst in the oxidation of bilirubin to biliverdin. This oxidation is characterized by a decrease in absorbance from 405—460 nm.
- Bilirubinometer: In this method, a bilirubinometer is used to read bilirubin concentration at 454 nm. The bilirubinometer is used as a direct spectrophotometric assay.
- Jendrassik-Grof: In this method, the coupling reaction of unconjugated bilirubin with the diazo reagent is accelerated with a caffeine-sodium benzoate mixture. This coupling reaction forms an azobilirubin complex, which can be used to determine bilirubin concentration in the sample. This method is the preferred method to use when determining serum bilirubin concentration, for it has a high recovery rate.
- Malloy-Evelyn: This particular method uses alcohol to dissolve unconjugated bilirubin. The unconjugated bilirubin then reacts with diazotized sulfanilic acid.

Gilbert's Syndrome

Gilbert's Syndrome is an inherited disorder that is characterized by the presence of an abnormal liver enzyme. This particular enzyme is necessary for the disposal of bilirubin. People with this syndrome have a problem with their hepatic uptake of bilirubin because this liver enzyme is abnormal. This syndrome is characterized by an increased level of unconjugated bilirubin, and a slightly elevated level of bilirubin in the blood. Mild jaundice is a side effect of this syndrome. The illness is often harmless, so often no treatment is required for people with Gilbert's Syndrome.

Dubin-Johnson Syndrome

In this syndrome, the transport of conjugated bilirubin is defective, and there is an impairment of the excretion of bilirubin in the bile. This leads to an increased level of conjugated (direct) bilirubin in serum, as well as an increased amount of bilirubin in the urine. There is no accompanying increase in the elevation of liver enzymes.

Crigler-Najjar Syndrome

This syndrome is characterized by an enzyme deficiency. The enzyme uridine diphosphate glucuronyl transferase is responsible for conjugating bilirubin. People with this syndrome are, therefore, unable to conjugate bilirubin, and an increased level of unconjugated bilirubin is displayed. Crigler-Najjar Syndrome is an hereditary disorder.

Ketone Bodies

Ketone bodies are substances containing ketone that are produced through a process called ketogenesis. In ketogenesis, ketone bodies are produced from the breaking down of fatty acids to produce energy. This degradation of fatty acids takes place in the cells of the liver. The ketone bodies are produced from acetyl coenzyme A (CoA) in the liver. Ketogenesis occurs when there are no or very few carbohydrates for the body to use to produce energy. This situation occurs most frequently due to starvation or uncontrolled Type I diabetes. Ketone bodies accumulate in the urine and the blood of such individuals. Examples of ketone bodies are acetone, acetoacetic acid, and beta-hydroxybutyric acid.

Hydrolysis

Hydrolysis is a chemical reaction of a molecule with water. Hydrolysis will result in the formation of new molecules. For example, if a molecule of disaccharide is hydrolyzed, the reaction will result in the formation of two monosaccharide molecules. Maltose, lactose, and sucrose are all disaccharides, and their hydrolysis each results in two monosaccharides. The hydrolysis of maltose results in two glucose molecules. The hydrolysis of a molecule of lactose results in the formation of a molecule of galactose and a molecule of glucose. And, finally, the hydrolysis of a molecule of sucrose results in the formation of a molecule of both fructose and a molecule of glucose.

Glucose Tolerance Test

A glucose tolerance test helps a physician understand and evaluate a patient's biological and chemical response to glucose. Glucose tolerance tests can be done with glucose administered to the patient either intravenously or orally. In a glucose tolerance test, blood glucose levels are taken at a fasting level, at one hour after glucose administration to the patient, at two hours after glucose administration, and again at three hours after glucose administration. Blood glucose levels can be taken at other times, as deemed necessary by the physician. The glucose tolerance test can be used to determine if a patient is diabetic, chemically speaking.

Glucose Tolerance Curve

A glucose tolerance curve of a non-diabetic patient shows a high blood glucose level at one hour after the administration of glucose, and the glucose level in the blood falls below the fasting glucose level at two hours after glucose administration. At three hours past glucose administration, the blood glucose levels in a non-diabetic patient should return to the fasting glucose level. The glucose tolerance curve of a diabetic patient will show above normal glucose levels, and glucose levels in the blood do not fall within the first two hours after glucose administration.

Tests for Carbohydrates and Reducing Substances

The most common **tests for carbohydrates** in the blood, urine, and spinal fluid are the glucose tests, but other forms of carbohydrates may be present. **Reducing substances** are carbohydrates that are present in a sample (such as blood, stool, urine, or spinal fluid) and help to diagnose a problem. For example, the presence of reducing substances in a stool specimen for a patient with diarrhea indicates that the diarrhea does not result from a parasitic or viral infection but rather an abnormality of carbohydrate excretion, such as lactase deficiency. Newborns are routinely screened for inborn errors of carbohydrate metabolism with reducing substance tests. If urine is negative for glucose but positive for reducing substances, then some other form of sugar (such as galactose, which indicates galactosemia) is present in the urine. Glucose is typically present in spinal fluid in lower amounts than in serum, and most reducing substances do not cross the blood-brain barrier.

Glycohemoglobin (A1C) Procedure

Glycohemoglobin (A1C) test measures hemoglobin A with a glucose molecule (glycated/glycosylated hemoglobin). When levels of glucose in the blood increase, the glucose binds to hemoglobin in the red blood cells in amounts proportional to the circulating glucose. Since the average life span of a red blood cell is 120 days with cells continuously dying and being replaced, the A1C test provides an average glucose level over about the previous 3 months:

- Normal value: 4% to 5.5%
- Prediabetes: 5.7% to 6.4%

Elevation: ≥6.5%

Critical results: >6.9%

Testing is done on a whole venous blood sample collected in a tube with anticoagulant, such as EDTA, or a fingerstick capillary specimen. The specimen may be stored under refrigeration at 4° to 8°C if testing is not carried out immediately. A glycohemoglobin analyzer is used to obtain laboratory results.

Serum Protein Electrophoresis and Protein Analysis

Total protein is measured with spectrophotometry and fractions of different plasma proteins by **serum protein electrophoresis** combined with immunoprecipitation (immunofixation electrophoresis, which divides the proteins according to size and charge). Plasma proteins include:

Total protein	0-5 days: 3.8-6.2 g/dL. Adult: 6-8 g/dL.	Increased: dehydration, monoclonal/polyclonal gammopathies, myeloma, sarcoidosis, chronic hepatic disease, leprosy, Waldenström macroglobulinemia.
		Decreased: Hypervolemia, burns, chronic alcoholism, liver disorders, kidney disorders, CHF, hyperthyroidism, malabsorption syndromes, neoplasms, pregnancy, starvation, prolonged immobilization.
Albumin	3.4-4.8 g/dL 55.5%	Increased: Dehydration, diarrhea, vomiting.
		Decreased: Renal disease, malnutrition, severe burns.
Alpha-1 globulin	0.2-0.4 g/dL 5.3%	Increased: Acute/chronic inflammatory diseases
		Decreased: Hereditary disease.
Alpha-2 globulin	0.4-0.8 g/dL 8.6%	Increased: Diabetes, pancreatitis, hemolysis.
		Decreased: Nephrotic syndrome, malignancies, inflammation, severe burn recovery period.
Beta globulin	0.5-1.0 g/dL 13.4%	Increased: Hyperlipoproteinemias, monoclonal gammopathies.
		Decreased: Hypo-?-lipoproteinemia, IgA deficiency.
Gamma globulin	0.6-1.2 g/dL 11% IgG—80% IgA—15% IgM—5% IgD—0.2% IgE—Trace.	Increased: Hepatic disease, chronic infections, autoimmune disorders, and lymphoproliferative disorders, multiple myeloma.
		Decreased: Immune deficiency/suppression.
		Note gamma globulin consists of 5 bands of immunoglobulins on electrophoresis: IgG, IgA, IgM, IgD, and IgE.

AFP Test

AFP stands for alpha-fetoprotein, and it is a protein that is produced by a fetus' liver. Alpha-fetoprotein can be detected in the mother's blood through a blood test. AFP reaches its highest concentration in the mother's blood between 12 and 15 weeks of gestation. Drawing the mother's blood at this time will thereby give the peak AFP released by the fetus. If the AFP levels in the mother's blood are found to be unusually high, there may be medical problems with the fetus, such as neural tube defects, including spina bifida, and anencephaly, or kidney problems. High AFP levels can also indicate twins. If the AFP levels are found to be unusually low, Down syndrome may be indicated. Ultrasound and amniocentesis can be used to confirm the results. Through amniocentesis, a sample of the amniotic fluid can be retrieved, and the AFP in the amniotic fluid can then be determined. Radioimmunoassay or immunoprecipitin methods can be used to quantify the amount of AFP present.

Biuret Procedure

The biuret procedure is used to determine the amount of protein in a sample. The procedure depends on the reaction between peptide linkages in the protein and copper ions in an alkaline solution. A reddish/violet color indicates the presence of peptide linkages, or proteins. The biuret procedure gives an accurate quantitation of the amount of total proteins found in a serum. A larger amount of proteins in a serum will have a larger quantity of peptide bonds, since all amino acids of proteins are joined by peptide bonds. A larger quantity of peptide bonds will lead to a more intense color produced by the reaction with the copper ions the biuret procedure. Typically, 4-6 peptide linkages will react/join with one copper ion complex. However, with a minimum of 2 peptide linkages available, the reaction will work, forming a reddish/violet colored product. Therefore, a tripeptide is the smallest protein that will react in the biuret procedure.

Kjeldahl Technique

The Kjeldahl technique is the reference method for quantifying the total protein found in a serum sample. The basis of the technique is the quantification of the number of peptide bonds present in the protein in the serum. In other words, the nitrogen content of the protein present is quantified. Through a reaction with sulfuric acid, the protein present undergoes digestion, which converts the nitrogen present in the protein to ammonium ions. The ammonium ion can then undergo distillation, which will give off ammonia, which can then be titrated. Or, the ammonium ion produced can be mixed with Nessler's reagent, which will form a colored product. This colored product can then be read spectrophotometrically. The Kjeldahl technique is thought to be too cumbersome to be used on a routine basis in the laboratory, but it is still considered to be the reference method for quantifying the total protein in a serum.

Endocrinology Concepts

The **endocrine system** includes numerous glands that have secretory cells but no ducts, so hormones produced are absorbed into the vascular system. Many hormones function under a negative feedback system: When the hormone level decreases, production increases, and when the hormone level increases, production is inhibited. Positive feedback occurs when the activity in an organ that is outside normal triggers release of hormone, such as increased release of oxytocin during childbirth and decrease in oxytocin after childbirth. Complex feedback involves interactions among a number of hormones, such as occurs with regulation of thyroid hormones. Some hormones are affected by nervous system reactions, such as when fear or anger triggers release of epinephrine. Some hormones cause the release of other hormones, such as thyrotropin-releasing hormone and prolactin-releasing hormone, while others inhibit hormones, such as prolactin-inhibiting hormone and somatostatin.

Production of Thyroid Hormones

The first step that needs to take place in order for the thyroid to produce its various hormones is for the thyroid to capture iodine from the rest of the body. Iodine can be captured from the gastrointestinal tract, for example. Once the thyroid has captured iodine, the iodine must then be activated. The activated form of iodine is called organic iodine. The organic, activated iodine then undergoes a process called organification. Organification is the process in which the iodine is attached to the tyrosine residues that are part of the protein thyroglobulin (TG). Thyroid stimulating hormone (TSH) then helps separate the iodinated tyrosines (the iodine coupled with the tyrosine) form the thyroglobulins. This forms T_3 (triiodothyronine) and T_4 (thyroxine), and these hormones are then released into the bloodstream. This separation and creation of triiodothyronine and thyroxine occurs on an as-needed basis in the body, regulated by TSH.

Effects of Vitamin D and PTH on Plasma Calcium Levels

When Vitamin D is hydroxylized (the addition of an OH group to the Vitamin D), a compound is produced that increases the absorption of phosphates and calcium in the intestines. Parathyroid hormone (PTH) is a hormone that helps maintain calcium levels in plasma. It helps move calcium from bones into the blood. PTH increases the creation of a particular derivative of Vitamin D, which causes an increase in the absorption of calcium in the intestines, and an increase in bone resorption. PTH production is shut off when normal calcium levels in the plasma are restored. PTH also helps regulate the amount of phosphorus.

Hormone Tests

Test	Normal values	Description
Adrenocorticotropic hormone (ACTH)	ACTH: 10-18 years: 6-55 pg/mL >18 years: 6-58 pg/mL	ACTH is produced in the anterior pituitary gland and released in response to increased hypothalamic-releasing factor. ACTH stimulates increased production of glucocorticoids (cortisol), androgens, and mineralocorticoids by the adrenals. ACTH is part of the hypothalamic-pituitary-adrenal axis. Increased: Addison disease (with low cortisol), Cushing disease (with high cortisol), carcinoid syndrome, congenital adrenal hyperplasia, depression, Nelson syndrome, septic shock/sepsis. Decreased: Adrenal adenoma or cancer, Cushing syndrome, steroid therapy.
	Stimulation with cosyntropin: Cortisol 18-20 mcg/dL or cortisol level increases 7 mcg/dL over baseline Stimulation with metyrapone (overnight): Cortisol <2 mcg/dL next day; ACTH >75 pg/mL	
	ACTH suppression with dexamethasone (overnight): Cortisol <1.87 mcg/dL next day	
Cortisol	8AM: 12-18 years—10-280 mcg/dL; >18 years—5-25 mcg/dL.	Primary glucocorticoid secreted by adrenal glands. Stimulates gluconeogenesis, serves as insulin antagonist, suppresses inflammatory response, and mobilizes proteins and fats. Test measures adrenal function.
	4 PM: 12-18 years—10-272 mcg/dL; >18 years—3-16 mcg/dL	
Dehydroepi-androsterone sulfate (DHEAS)	Varies by age, gender, and Tanner stage: Male: 3-6 years: 0-50 mcg/dL 15-19 years: 88-483 mcg/dL 20-29 years: 280-640 mcg/dL 60-69 years: 42-290 mcg/dL Female: 3-6 years: 0-50 mcg/dL 15-19 years: 63-373 mcg/dL 20-29 years: 65-380 mcg/dL 60-69 years: 13-130 mcg/dL	Metabolite of primary adrenal androgen (DHEA), synthesized in adrenals and testes. Can convert into testosterone or estradiol. Increased: Cushing syndrome, anovulation, hirsutism, polycystic ovarian syndrome, adrenal tumors (virilizing), ACTH-producing tumors. Decreased: Addison disease, hyperlipidemia, pregnancy, psoriasis, psychosis.
Parathyroid hormone (PTH)	2-20 years: 9-52 pg/mL	Produced in parathyroid glands and released in response to low calcium levels to mobilize movement of calcium from bones into blood. Increased: Hyperparathyroidism, fluorosis, Zollinger-Ellison syndrome, pseudogout. Decreased: Hypoparathyroidism, hyperparathyroidism (associated with increased serum calcium), sarcoidosis.
	>20 years: 10-065 pg/mL	

ADH: 0-18 years 0.5-1.5 pg/mL >18 years 0-5 pg/mL Correlated with serum osmolality: 270-280 mOsm/kg—<1.5 pg/mL 280-285 mOsm/kg—<2.5 pg/mL 285-290 mOsm/kg—1-5 pg/mL 290-295 mOsm/kg—2-7 pg/mL 295-300 mOsm/kg—4-12 pg/mL	Produced in hypothalamus, stored in posterior pituitary gland, and released with decreased blood volume or increased serum osmolality. Causes the kidneys to reabsorb more water to maintain proper osmolality and fluid balance. Increased: Brain tumor, CNS disorders, hypovolemia, Guillain-Barré, diabetes insipidus (DI) (nephrogenic), SIADH. Decreased: Hypervolemia, nephrotic syndrome, DI (pituitary), pituitary surgery, psychogenic polydipsia.

Aldosterone: 11-15 years supine 2-22 ng/dL 11-15 years upright 4-48 ng/dL >15 years supine 3-16 ng/dL >15 years upright 7-30 ng/dL	Mineralocorticoid produced by adrenal glands in response to increased potassium, decreased sodium, or decreased blood volume. Release triggered by angiotensin II. Helps to regulate sodium and potassium levels. Increased: Adenomas (with decreased renin), cardiac failure, COPD, cirrhosis, diuretic/laxative abuse, hypovolemia, nephrotic syndrome, starvation, toxemia. Decreased: (With hypertension) Addison disease; (Without hypertension) alcohol intoxication, diabetes, Turner syndrome.

Thyroid Function Tests

Thyroid-stimulating hormone (TSH)	0.4-6.15 μg/U/mL	Released from pituitary gland, triggered by thyrotropin-releasing hormone (hypothalamus). Stimulates thyroid to produce triiodothyronine (T3) and thyroxine (T4), which regulate metabolism. Increased: Hypothyroidism. Decreased: Hyperthyroidism.
Free T3	17-20 ng/dL	Regulates cell metabolic rate, cell growth, and cell differentiation. Increased: Hyperthyroidism, high altitude, T3 toxicosis. Decreased: Hypothyroidism, malnutrition, chronic disease (non-thyroid), late pregnancy.
T3 resin uptake	25-35%	Test to estimate amounts of free T3, T4, and TBG. Increased: Hyperthyroidism. Decreased: Hypothyroidism.
T4 total	4.5-11.5 μg/dL	May be affected by levels of TBG. Increased: Iodine toxicity, psychiatric disorder, hepatitis, hyperthyroidism, obesity, thyrotoxicosis (Graves') and thyrotoxicosis factitia. Decreased: Low TBG level, hypothyroidism, panhypopituitarism, excessive exercise.
Free T4	0.9-1.7 ng/dL	Precursor to T3, not affected by levels of TBG. Increased: Hyperthyroidism. Decreased: Hypothyroidism.
Thyroxine-binding globulin (TBG)	0-50 ng/mL	Protein that transports thyroid hormones. Increased: Thyroid cancer, Graves diseases, thyroiditis, thyrotoxicosis. Decreased: Thyrotoxicosis factitia, administration of thyroid hormones, and congenital athyrosis (in neonates).

24-Hour Urine Endocrinology Tests

Thyroid hormone test	T3: 15-18 years 1.1-2.7 nmol/L >18 years 0.9-2.4 nmol/L	Urine levels may be higher than serum because serum levels vary during the day.
	T4: 14-17 years 5-9.8 mcg/dL ≥18 years 4.8-10.4 mcg/dL	Urine levels may be higher than serum.
	Selenium ≤200 mcg/L with creatinine correction <25 mcg/g	Selenium converts T4 into T3. Levels may be higher or lower with cancer. Levels are decreased in children, older adults, and pregnant women.

5-Hydroxyindoleacetic acid (5-HIAA)	2-10 years <8 mg/g creatinine >10 years <6 mg/d	Product of serotonin metabolism. Used to measure serotonin level. Increased: carcinoid and neuroendocrine tumors, cystic fibrosis, celiac disease. Decreased: renal disease, phenylketonuria

Reproductive Hormone Tests

Follicle-stimulating hormone (FSH)	Male: 1.4-15.5 IU/mL. Female: Varies according to cycle, increases during ovulation: 7.2-17.2 IU/mL. Postmenopausal: 19-100 IU/mL.	Used to manage/diagnose menstrual problems, infertility, abnormal sexual development. Increased: Alcoholism, Klinefelter syndrome, hypogonadism, Turner syndrome, precocious puberty. Decreased: Anorexia nervosa, hemochromatosis, polycystic ovary disease, pregnancy, sickle cell anemia, hypothalamic disorder.
Luteinizing hormone (LH)	Male; 0.5-1.9 IU/mL. Female, varies according to cycle, increases during ovulation: 21.9-80. Postmenopausal: 14.2-52.3 IU/mL.	Used to assess gonadal function, fertility issues, treatment response. Increased: Gonadal disorders, menopause. Decreased: Anorexia nervosa, malnutrition, hypothalamic/pituitary dysfunction, stress.
17-ketosteroids	Varies widely according to age, gender, and Tanner stage	Used to evaluate androgen excess, adrenal tumors, congenital adrenal hyperplasia, and (in females) infertility, amenorrhea, and excess hair growth. Increased: Cushing syndrome, polycystic ovary syndrome, hirsutism, anovulation. Decreased: Addison disease, adrenal insufficiency, hyperlipidemia, pregnancy, psoriasis, psychosis.
Estrogen (estriol, estradiol, and estrone)	Estriol: Levels vary	Measured during pregnancy, evident by 9 weeks.
	Estradiol: Levels vary by gender, age, menstrual cycle, and menopause	Used to diagnose infertility associated with tumor or ovarian failure.
	Estrone—primary source of estrogen after menopause. Males: 10-60 pg/mL Adult females: 17-200 pg/mL Postmenopausal females: 7-40 pg/mL.	Estrone—used to assess estrogen level in post-menopausal women and to assess estrogen levels in males and females with ovarian, testicular, and adrenal malignancies.

Testosterone	Varies by age and gender: Male 8-10 y: 0-25 ng/dL Male 13-15 y: 15-500 ng/dL Male >15 y: 241-827 ng/dL Female 8-10 y: 0-30 ng/dL Female 13-15 y: 0-50 ng/dL Female >15 y: 15-70 ng/dL	Used to assess disorders of puberty and infertility and gonadal/adrenal function. Increased: Adrenal hyperplasia, adrenocortical tumors, hirsutism, hyperthyroidism, idiopathic sexual precocity, polycystic ovaries, testicular tumors, virilizing ovarian tumors. Decreased: Anovulation, cryptorchidism, alcoholism, impotence, Klinefelter syndrome, myotonic dystrophy, hypogonadism, hypopituitarism, uremia.

Determining Inorganic Phosphate Concentration in Serum

The basis of this determination is reacting a deproteinized serum with a molybdate reagent. The phosphate in the serum, once reacting with the molybdate reagent, will form a phosphomolybdate compound. This compound can then be combined with a reducing agent to form molybdenum blue. The resulting molybdenum blue can then be measured in the laboratory spectrophotometrically to determine the inorganic phosphate concentration in the serum.

Components of Total Anion Content of Serum in Healthy Adults

The highest concentration of the total anion content of a serum is of chloride, followed by bicarbonate. The next highest concentration is that of negatively charged proteins. These proteins make up approximately 16 mmol of charge per liter. Lactate has the next highest concentration, and finally, ketone bodies, such as acetate, make up the smallest concentration of the total anion content of a serum.

Water-Soluble and Fat-Soluble Vitamins

Thiamin, ascorbic acid, niacin, and riboflavin are all water-soluble vitamins. Vitamin A, Vitamin D, Vitamin E, and vitamin K are all fat soluble.

Vitamin K at Birth

Vitamin K is a very important vitamin because it is related to proper clotting of the blood. It helps form prothrombin to make a clot. If there is a lack of Vitamin K, there will be a corresponding decrease in the production of prothrombin. Adults with decreased prothrombin have increased PT/PTT times, broken capillaries and bruising. Vitamin K is synthesized in the intestines of newborns, and since their intestinal flora are often underdeveloped at birth, there may not be enough Vitamin K synthesized. This can lead to hemorrhagic disease or navel bleeding in newborn babies. An intramuscular injection of Vitamin K at birth can help ward off such problems by supplying the newborn with the Vitamin K that he/she needs until the newborn is able to synthesize enough Vitamin K independently.

Pharmacokinetics

Pharmacokinetics include the route of administration, the absorption, the dosage, the frequency of administration, the distribution, and the serum levels achieved over time. The drug's rate of clearance (elimination) and doses needed to ensure therapeutic benefit must be considered. Most drugs are cleared through the kidneys, with water-soluble compounds excreted more readily than protein-soluble compounds. Volume of distribution (IV drug dose divided by plasma concentration) determines the rate at which the drug passes into tissue. Drug distribution depends on the degree of protein binding and ion trapping that takes place. Effect-site equilibrium is the time between administration of a drug and clinical effect (the point at which the drug reaches the appropriate receptors) and must be considered when determining dose, time, and frequency of drugs. The bioavailability of drugs may vary, depending upon the degree of metabolism that takes place before the drug reaches its site of action.

Pharmacodynamics

Pharmacodynamics relates to biological effects (therapeutic or adverse) of drug administration over time. Drug transport, absorption, means of elimination, and half-life must all be considered when determining effects. Responses may include continuous responses, such as blood pressure variations, or dichotomous response in which an event either occurs or does not (such as death). Information from pharmacodynamics provides feedback to modify medication dosage (pharmacokinetics). Drugs provide biological effects primarily by interacting with receptor sites (specific protein molecules) in the cell membrane. Receptors include voltage-sensitive ion channels (sodium, chloride, potassium, and calcium channels), ligand-gated ion channels, and transmembrane receptors. Agonist drugs exert effects after binding with a receptor while antagonist drugs bind with a receptor but have no effects, so they can block agonists from binding. The total number of receptors may vary, upregulating or downregulating in response to stimuli (such as drug administration). Dose-response curves show the relationship between the amount of drug given and the resultant plasma concentration and biological effects.

Toxicological Tests

Screening tests determine if classes of drugs (such as opioids) are present. **Confirmatory tests** determine if a false negative or positive has occurred and identifies specific drugs. **Toxicological tests** assess the presence or level of drugs or other substances in blood, urine, hair, or saliva and therapeutic drug monitoring (TDM).

Antidepressants	Antidepressant drug profile (urine) shows presence of multiple antidepressants. TDM used for specific drugs.
Antibiotics	Aminoglycoside test used to monitor drug levels 6-144 hours after dose. Specific TDM for different antibiotics.
Beta blockers	BB panel tests for multiple drugs. Hypoglycemia is common with BB toxicity.
Calcium channel blockers	TDM. With toxicity, multiple other tests (glucose, electrolytes, blood gases, ECG) are needed. Hyperglycemia is common with CCB toxicity.

Therapeutic Drug Monitoring

Plasma drug levels are used for **therapeutic drug monitoring** because, although plasma is often not the site of action, plasma levels correlate well with therapeutic and toxic responses to most drugs. The therapeutic range of a drug is that between the minimum effective concentration (level at which there is no therapeutic benefit) and the toxic concentration (level at which toxic effects occur). To achieve drug plateau (steady state), the drug half-life (time needed to decrease drug concentration by 50%) must be considered. Most drugs reach plateau with administration equal to 4 half-lives and completely eliminate a drug in 5 half-lives. Because drug levels fluctuate, peak (highest drug concentration) and trough (lowest drug concentration) levels may be monitored. Samples for trough levels are taken immediately prior to administration of another dose while peak samples are taken at various times, depending on the average peak time of the specific drug, which may vary from 30 minutes to about 2 hours after administration.

Barbiturates

Barbiturates are a class of drug that acts as a depressant or a body sedative. These drugs depress the activity of the nervous system, including parts of the brain. Barbiturates depress the functions of all body tissues to some extent. Barbiturates lower blood pressure and respiratory rate. Small doses of barbiturates induce sleepiness and drowsiness, while high doses act as anesthetics, and overdoses can even cause coma and death. The barbiturates are differentiated according to their activity level: Long-acting, intermediate-acting, short-acting, and very short-acting barbiturates. The long-acting barbiturates have increased therapeutic duration when compared to the shorter acting barbiturates. Long-acting barbiturates require higher doses to be toxic. Some examples of barbiturates include: Phenobarbital (long- acting), amobarbital (intermediate-acting), pentobarbital (short- acting), and thiopental sodium (very short-acting).

Drugs of Abuse

Drug of abuse is a term used for any substance used in a way or quantity beyond the recommendation or without any medical oversight. Substances tested can include amphetamines, barbiturates, benzodiazepines, cannabinoids, opiates, tricyclic antidepressants, oxycodone, oxymorphone, MDMA (ecstasy), cocaine, PCP (angel dust), methadone, and metabolites associated with each.

Tests for Detection

The detection of drugs of abuse is part of the field of toxicology. There are several material sources from the body that can be used to achieve varying degrees of specificity in detection including blood, urine, saliva, hair, and sweat. Urine is a common material for detecting substances as it can have the strongest signal, but over a small time-window. Conversely, hair has a much longer detection window, but the signal is very weak. Regardless of the material used, testing is usually comprised of two independent methodologies to confirm results. Laboratory personnel often use a screening process to obtain a qualitative pass/fail result in conjunction with a more robust quantitative measurement of concentration. The most common screening methods are ELISA and test strips. Quantitative methods utilize gas or liquid chromatography (separating) and mass spectrometry (measuring) to confirm any initial screening results.

Isoenzyme Electrophoresis and Hemoglobin Electrophoresis

Isoenzyme electrophoresis separates enzymes into components with different molecular structure (isoenzymes) according to size and charge. For example lactase dehydrogenase (LDH) has 5 isoenzymes, numbered consecutively, but LDH1 is found in the heart muscle and increases with an MI while LDH5 increases with liver disease. Creatine kinase has three isoenzymes: CK-BB in brain and lungs, CK-MG in cardiac muscle, and CK-MM in skeletal muscle. Alkaline phosphatase has 12 isoenzymes, including the bone, liver and the liver fractions, which are most important for diagnoses.

Hemoglobin electrophoresis		
Hemoglobin (identifies normal and abnormal forms of Hgb)	Hgb A: >95%	Most common form of Hgb.
	Hgb A2: 1.5-3.7%	Increased: Hyperthyroidism, sickle cell trait, and β-thalassemia and megaloblastic anemia. Decreased: Iron deficiency anemia, sideroblastic anemia, erythroleukemia.
	Hgb F (fetal): Newborn: 70-77% 6 mo: 3-7% Adult: <2%	Increased: Aplastic anemia, anemia of blood loss, leukemia, myeloproliferative disorders, pernicious anemia, thalassemias, sickle cell disease.
	Hgb D, E, H, S, C: Presence indicates abnormality	Found in inherited hemoglobinopathies. Increased E: thalassemia-like disorder. Increased: Sickle cell disease. Increased H: α-thalassemia.

Enzyme-Multiplied Immunoassay Technique

The enzyme-multiplied immunoassay technique (EMIT) is used to determine the concentration of a particular drug in a serum sample by using an enzyme label. First, an antibody that is specific to the drug in question is added to the sample. Secondly, a coenzyme and a substrate for the enzyme label are then added to the serum sample. Finally, the free labeled antigen (the enzyme labeled drug) is added to the serum sample. The enzyme labeled drug that has been added to the serum then competes with the particular drug in question that is already present in the serum sample for binding sites on the antibody that had been added. When the enzyme labeled drug binds to the antibody, decreased enzyme activity is exhibited, resulting in the free enzyme labeled drug being the only thing that can react with the substrate and the coenzyme. Enzyme activity is measured at 340 nm, and it is directly proportional to the amount of the particular drug in the serum. The higher the concentration of the particular drug in the serum, the higher the amount of enzyme activity.

Reinsch Test

The Reinsch Test is a laboratory test used to determine the presence of heavy metals in a sample, often urine. In this particular test, the urine sample is dissolved in a solution of hydrochloric acid (HCl). After the urine is dissolved, a strip of copper is placed into the solution. If a heavy metal is present, the copper strip will develop a colored coating. A silver coating may indicate the presence of mercury, while a blackish/blue color (or another dark color) may indicate the presence of another heavy metal, such as antimony, arsenic, bismuth, selenium, or thallium. The test is a rapid one, and is good for a quick, initial screening. However, the findings of this test should be confirmed with other laboratory techniques.

Trinder Reaction

The Trinder Reaction is used most often to determine the presence of salicylate in the urine. A solution containing ferric chloride is added to the urine sample in question. An iron complex will form between the ferric chloride and the salicylate, if salicylate is present. This reaction will turn the solution a purple color. The test is very rapid, and this is one of its positive points. However, the test has the possibility for false positive results as well. A purple color will also be produced if any enol or phenol is present in the urine, as well as if the patient has an elevated urine bilirubin level of 1 mg/dL or greater.

Fetal Wellness Tests

Lecithin/sphingomyelin (L/S) ratio: The ratio of the phospholipids lecithin and sphingomyelin (two components of surfactant) changes during pregnancy with L/S ratio at 0.5:1 early in pregnancy, 1:1 at 30-32 weeks, and 2:1 at 35 weeks. This test is not accurate if the amniotic fluid contains blood or meconium. **Alpha-fetoprotein (AFT)** is a protein produced by the yolk sac for the first 6 weeks of gestation and then by the fetal liver. Cutoff levels have been established for each week of gestation, with peak levels at about week 15. The test is used primarily to detect neural tube defects (NTDs), which develop in the first trimester. AFT can be measured in amniotic fluid or maternal serum. **Delta 450** is an amniotic bilirubin scan, usually done only with fetal transfusion because it requires amniocentesis. **Fibronectin** (an adhesive glycoprotein that adheres fetal membrane to placenta) is measured in vaginal secretions and is present early in pregnancy and near term (after week 35). Earlier detection may indicate preterm labor.

Metabolism of Purines, Formation of Uric Acid, and Tests for Gout

Gout (metabolic arthritis) is a group of conditions associated with a defect of purine metabolism, resulting in hyperuricemia with oversecretion of uric acid, decreased excretion of uric acid, or a combination. Purine is ingested in food, especially meats. Increased uric acid levels can cause monosodium urate crystal depositions in the joints, resulting in severe articular and periarticular inflammation. With chronic gout, sodium urate crystals, called tophi, accumulate in peripheral body areas, such as the great toe (75%), ankle, knee, hands, and ears. Assessment is through uric acid levels:

- Normal values: Male 4.4 to 7.6 mg/dL, Female 2.3 to 6.6 mg/dL.

Crystals may begin to form with levels >7. Testing is carried out on 1 mL serum collected in a red- or tiger-capped or heparinized green-capped tube. If the patient is receiving rasburicase, the specimen must be collected in a pre-chilled heparinized green-capped tube and transported in ice slurry. Analysis is done with spectrophotometry. A joint fluid test with microscopic analysis may also be carried out with aspirated synovial fluid.

REFRACTOMETERS

Refractometers are used to measure fluid concentration by assessing light refraction through a prism. Refractometers vary in size and sophistication (simple handheld devices to more complex digital devices), so procedures may vary. Generally, the instrument is calibrated with water before the sample is tested. Testing:

- Turn on equipment.
- Clean prism with cotton ball and ethanol or according to manufacturer's guidelines.
- Place sample on prism or in sample well and secure prism.
- Look through the eyepiece, adjust as needed for manual equipment.
- Read results expressed in Brix (1 degree Brix = 1 g sucrose in 100 g solution), refractive index (degree to which the light is bent), and/or specific gravity. Digital equipment provides a read-out.
- Note: Tables are available that provide the refractive index for most common materials

Refractometers may be used to assess urine specific gravity, serum copper sulfate, and serum protein. Sample temperature must be maintained within a prescribed temperature range for some types of refractometers.

BILIRUBIN AND GASTRIC SECRETIONS FOR OCCULT BLOOD

Bilirubin	Uncoagulated blood sample allowed to clot at room temperature and then centrifuged and supernatant separated immediately for examination. Direct: Dilute sample by mixing 1 mL with 4 mL saline. Label 2 tubes for direct bilirubin (DB) and serum blank (SB). Place 1 mL diluted serum and 2 mL 0.05 hydrochloric acid in each tube. Place 0.5 mL Diazo II reagent in DB and in exactly 60 seconds add 0.1 mL ascorbic acid, mix, and add 1.5 mL alkaline tartrate and read color results in 5-10 minutes. To tube SB, place 0.5 mL Diazo I reagent, 0.5 mL ascorbic acid, and 1.5 mL alkaline tartrate, and mix to use as serum blank.
Occult blood (gastric)	Sample is applied to paper reagent strip coated with guaiac, which changes color to blue in the presence of blood within 1 minute. The sample may also be applied to a slide (thin smear), which is examined microscopically.

BODY FLUID CYTOCENTRIFUGATION

Cytocentrifugation ("cytospin") uses a special centrifuge with slide holders that have attached funnels to hold body fluid that has been mixed with a medium in prescribed amounts. The process is able to concentrate cells that occur in small numbers in a sample. During centrifugation (usually at about 500 rpm for about 5 minutes), the fluid is wicked into a filter and onto a slide in a thin monolayer. Albumin (11% or 22%) may be added to serous fluids to preserve morphology as centrifugation may result in some distortion (although clumping patterns and ratio of nucleus to cytoplasm are unchanged). Albumin should not be added to synovial fluid. Cells in body fluids are similar to those in peripheral blood, and morphology is similar but counts are usually less. Once the slide is prepared, staining may be done to facilitate evaluation.

SEMEN ANALYSIS

These are the parameters for a semen analysis: General color and clarity of the semen should be a grayish-white and translucent. The pH should be between 7.3 and 7.8, and the viscosity of the semen (the resistance of the semen to flow) should get a rating of one on a scale of one to four. The volume of the entire ejaculate should be between two and five milliliters. Coagulation and liquefaction should occur within 30 minutes of collecting the sample. The motility of the sperm, or the percentage of sperm present that are moving, should be about 60% or higher. The percentage of sperm that are moving forward (forward progression) should be at least 50% or higher. The sperm count should be a minimum of 40 million sperm per total ejaculate. At least 30% of the sperm present should have a normal morphology, with no double or deformed tails or heads.

Use of Amniotic Fluid Measurements in Laboratory

The lecithin/sphingomyelin ratio in the amniotic fluid is a good indicator for the lung maturity of the fetus. Via amniocentesis, a sample of surfactant in the amniotic fluid is removed. The lecithin/sphingomyelin ratio is then calculated. If the ratio is less than 2, then the fetal lungs are not producing enough surfactant, and this is an indicator that the fetal lungs may be immature (wet). Determining the lecithin/sphingomyelin ratio is very important because it can help predict and/or prevent fetal respiratory distress after birth.

The concentrations of creatinine and urea nitrogen in amniotic fluid are useful for helping determine if amniotic fluid is contaminated with any maternal urine. Using amniocentesis, a sample of amniotic fluid is extracted from the mother's uterus. Because creatinine and urea nitrogen concentrations in the mother's urine are much greater (on the order of ten to fifty times greater) than those concentrations in amniotic fluid, an unexpected high concentration of creatinine and/or urea nitrogen in the amniotic fluid can indicate contamination of the amniotic fluid with maternal urine, often by bladder puncture.

Determining Concentration of Particular Cells Using the Hemocytometer

Use a Neubauer-ruled hemocytometer to manually count blood cells or other microscopic particles in blood. The hemocytometer is a glass microscope slide with rectangular indentations that create a chamber with a depth of 0.1 mm. This chamber is scored with a series of perpendicular lines that form a grid (fields). Dilute a blood sample and pipette 10 microliters inside the chamber. Cover it with a glass coverslip. The diluted sample spreads across the chamber. Wait 10 minutes for cells to settle. Examine the chamber at 10x magnification under the microscope. Differentiate and count the cells in 9 large fields. Report the total WBC count per cubic millimeter as the (number of cells counted X10 X100) /9.

Schilling Test

The Schilling test is used to determine if a deficiency in gastric intrinsic factor (IF) exists in a patient. In this test, the patient takes an oral radioactive isotope of Vitamin B_{12} labeled with cobalt, then completes a 24-hour urine collection. The isotope needs intrinsic factor in order to be adequately absorbed by the intestine, and then it should be excreted in the patient's urine. However, if the isotope collected in the urine is abnormally low (below 7%), not enough intrinsic factor is present. So the test is repeated, but this time with intrinsic factor added to the isotope, and the amount of the isotope in the urine is determined again. If the amount of isotope in the second urine is at a normal level, then the patient is said to have a deficiency in the gastric intrinsic factor. This results in pernicious anemia, in which the patient has difficulty absorbing vitamin B_{12}. Pernicious anemia is common among vegans who have eaten no animal products for more than five years.

Measuring Hemoglobin

Hemoglobin can be measured in the laboratory using cyanide reagents. To measure hemoglobin, mix the blood sample with a solution containing potassium ferricyanide. The potassium ferricyanide oxidizes the iron found in the hemoglobin to its ferric state. Once its iron is oxidized, the hemoglobin is referred to as methemoglobin. Add potassium cyanide to the methemoglobin to form cyanmethemoglobin. Measure the cyanmethemoglobin using spectrophotometric techniques. The hemoglobin concentration present is proportional to the optical density of the cyanmethemoglobin formed in this reaction. The reagent used to measure hemoglobin used to be called Drabkin's reagent, but it is now called cyanmethemoglobin (HiCN) reagent.

Osmotic Fragility Test

The osmotic fragility test is based on the ability of a red blood cell to hold up when exposed to variances in salt concentration of a solution. Certain cells, such as spherocytes (spherical shaped red blood cells), will swell and eventually burst (hemolyze) as the salt concentration in the solution decreases. As the salt concentration decreases, more water will enter the red blood cell because of the principle of osmosis. If the cell has accepted the maximum amount of water that it can, but water is still trying to enter the red blood cell and the pressure inside the cell keeps increasing, the cell will burst, releasing hemoglobin (hemolysis). The reason that spherocytes are susceptible to hemolyzing in this test is because they have a low ratio of surface area to volume, as opposed to normal erythrocytes that are donut-shaped. Spherocytes are osmotically fragile—not as resilient to pressure as are normally shaped erythrocytes.

COMPLETE BLOOD COUNT

A complete blood count, or CBC, consists of a white blood cell count, a red blood cell count, a platelet count, hemoglobin and mean cell volume, all of which are usually automated. A white blood cell differential is also performed manually on a smear if the doctor requests a diff. Hematocrit tubes are centrifuged to find the percentage of red cells by volume. Red blood cell indices are calculated using hemoglobin and hematocrit values with the red blood cell count. A complete blood cell count is performed to help diagnose a person with an infection, anemia, bleeding, leukemia, and some poisons. Pre-operative patients have a precautionary CBC before surgery. Complete blood cell counts can help a doctor check the progress of treatments for anemia, and the effectiveness of radiation and chemotherapy on cancers.

BONE MARROW ASPIRATION PROCEDURE AND TOUCH PREPS

Bone marrow aspiration is usually done in the posterior superior (most common) or anterior superior iliac crest (or tibia for infants <1 year). Patients are placed in lateral decubitus or prone position, and adults receive local anesthesia and pediatric patients receive general anesthesia. Using aseptic technique, the procedure includes:

- Infiltrating local anesthetic (10 mL/10% lidocaine).
- Making small surgical incision.
- Inserting aspiration needle through incision and into bone (turning back and forth to advance) until entering bone marrow cavity and then aspirating 0.3 mL bone marrow.
- Immediately preparing slide or storing marrow in EDTA tube.
- Removing needle, applying pressure, and applying dressing.

Touch prep (to have 6 slides with morphological imprints of bone marrow biopsy):

- Lay out 6 slides and place the marrow core on one.
- Use a cover slide to roll the core across the first slide.
- Use the second cover slide to roll the core across the second slide.
- Use the third cover slide to roll the core across the third slide.
- For aspirate, use smear technique (results in 1 slide), pull technique (2 slides), or lift technique (2 slides) (least effective method.)

INTERFERING FACTORS/SUBSTANCES IN HEMOGLOBIN MEASUREMENT

Tourniquet in place for >60 seconds	May increase levels up to 5%. Avoid extended use of tourniquet.
Rapid blood loss	Hgb may stay within normal parameters initially, so use other assessments.
Transfusion, recent	Hgb may remain unchanged initially, so be aware.
Cold agglutinins	May increase MCHC and decrease RBC count and hgb. Warm blood products, administer warm saline instead of plasma and recheck.
Positional change	Hgb may increase when upright and decrease when declining, so note position.

Hemolysis	Clotted or hemolyzed specimens should be rejected and specimen redrawn.
Lipids	May increase Hgb, MCV and MCHC. Administer warm saline instead of plasma and recheck and manually correct utilizing appropriate formula.
Copper deficiency	May decrease Hgb. Provide appropriate treatment.
RBC abnormalities	Some disorders, such as sickle cell disease, cause anemia and low Hgb. Treatment is usually provided to reach target Hgb.
Drugs	May increase or decrease Hgb. Note patient's medications.

WBC COUNT AND DIFFERENTIAL

Automated methods of determining the **WBC count and differential** (and other cells) include hematology analyzers: Electrical impedance (blood cells pass through 2 electrodes and the impedance changes according to cell volume) and flow cytometry (uses lasers and reagents to pass blood cells through a laser beam to determine cell morphology). Manual method:

1. Gently mix blood with Turk diluent and wait 2 minutes for hemolysis to complete. 20× dilution is standard but high WBC counts may require up to 100× dilution.
2. Fill counting chamber by capillary and place on microscope stage.
3. Focus on one "W" marked area and count the cells in each square (cells blue with dark nucleus).
4. Count both sides of chamber and average counts of both sides (4 sq mm area).
5. Apply formula: (#WBC counted/area counted × fluid depth) × dilution.

For the differential count, prepare a blood smear, stain the smear, examine with microscope under oil immersion objective, and count each cell until 100 cells counted, noting any abnormalities. Note blast or immature cells. Nucleated red blood cells observed are counted separately.

WHITE BLOOD CELL (LEUKOCYTE) COUNT

Differential	Normal	Changes
Total WBC	4,800-10,000	Increased (10,000+): Severe infection. (See differential for other.) Decreased (<4000): Viral infection, autoimmune disorders.
Total neutrophils	2.7-6.5 4.5-11.1%	Increased: Infections, injuries, inflammatory disorders, lymphocytic leukemias. Decreased: Bacterial infections, viral infections, aplastic anemia, autoimmune disorders, splenomegaly, chemotherapy, toxin exposure.
Immature neutrophils (bands)	0.1-0.3 1-3%	Increased: Infection, acute hemorrhage, acute hemolysis, malignancies, metabolic disorders, myelocytic leukemia, tissue necrosis, toxin ingestion. Decreased: Addison disease, anaphylaxis, anorexia nervosa, SLE, viral infection, folate deficiency, thyrotoxicosis.
Segmented neutrophils	2.5-6.2 50-62%	Increased: Acute, localized, or systemic bacterial infections.
Eosinophils	0.05-0.5 0-3%	Decreased: Stress and acute infection.
Basophils	0-0.1 0-1%	Decreased: Acute stage of infection.
Lymphocytes	1.5-3.7 25-40%	Increased: Some viral and bacterial infections, Addison disease, lymphocytic leukemia, lymphomas, myeloma, lymphosarcoma, ulcerative colitis. Decreased: Burns, Hodgkin's disease, pernicious anemia, radiation, septicemia, corticosteroids, bone marrow failure, immunosuppressive drugs, thrombocytopenia purpura, transfusion reaction.

Differential	Normal	Changes
Monocytes	0.2-0.4 3-7%	Increased: Recovery stage of acute infection, cirrhosis, hemolytic anemias, Hodgkin's disease, sarcoidosis, radiation, polycythemia vera, collagen diseases.

Thrombocyte Maturation Series and Blood Smear for Platelets

The **thrombocyte maturation series** includes:

- Hemocytoblast (able to produce all cell types)
- Myeloid stem cells
- Megakaryoblast (21-50 μm) with irregular-shaped nucleus.
- Promegakaryocyte (20-80 μm) with 2-4 small nucleoli.
- Megakaryocyte (≤100 μm) with multi-lobed nucleus.
- Thrombocyte

Count increased in polycythemia vera, RA, acute infections, anemias, cirrhosis, chronic leukemia, splenectomy, TB, ulcerative colitis, and trauma. Count decreased in aplastic anemia, megaloblastic anemia, iron-deficiency anemia, idiopathic thrombocytopenia, severe hemorrhage, bone marrow replacement, radiation, multiple infections, lymphoma, aplastic anemia

Blood smear for platelets may be carried out if the automated blood count shows an abnormally high or low. For the smear, a slide is treated with a stain and a drop of blood spread thinly across the slide. A microscopic examination or digital analyzer may be used to analyze the smear and determine the size and shape of the platelets. For example, if the platelets are exceptionally large ("giant") (the size of RBCs), this may be an indication of myeloproliferative neoplasm or immune thrombocytopenic purpura. A blood smear can also help to differentiate clumps of platelets from enlarged platelets.

Sources of Error and Corrective Actions for Platelet Counts

Platelet counts (150,000-450,000) are usually done electronically, but the tendency of platelets to clump and their small size can interfere with accurate counts. Accuracy decreases with low platelet numbers (around 100,000), sometimes causing analyzers to overestimate the counts by up to 30%. Abnormal findings:

- Falsely decreased counts may result from inadequate anticoagulation, platelet clumping, presence of giant platelets, and platelet adherence to neutrophils (satellitism resulting from antibodies). The solution may be to use a fresh fingerstick sample for a blood film. Manual counting may be necessary for giant platelets, which may be miscounted as RBCs. For platelet aggregation caused by EDTA, solutions include adding more EDTA, adding kanamycin (20 mg), collecting a sample in citrate rather than EDTA, or using a fingerstick sample with no anticoagulant.
- Falsely elevated counts may result from microcytosis, fragmentation of leukocytes, and presence of cryoglobulins. The solution may be to do a phase contrast microscopic examination or estimation based on a blood film. All abnormal counts should be confirmed with a second test.

Body Fluid Analysis, Counts, and Related Morphology

Cerebrospinal Fluid and Synovial Fluid

Cerebrospinal fluid is similar to plasma, from which it is derived, but with lower levels of protein and some electrolyte differences. Composition:

Appearance: clear with no clot	Protein: Myelin basic—<4.0 ng/mL, IgG—3.4 mg/dL
Electrolytes: Na 138 mEq/L, K 2.8 mEq/L, Ca, 2.1 mEq/L, Mg 2-2.5 mEq/L, Cl 119 mEq/L	WBC count: 0-1 mo.—0-30 cells/mm^3, 5-adult—0-5 cells/mm^3. No abnormal cells. RBC count: 0
Glucose: Infant/child—60-80 mg/dL, Adult—40-70 mg/dL.	Lactic acid: Neonate—10-60 mg/dL, Adult—<25.2 mg/dL

Synovial fluid composition:

Appearance: clear to pale yellow, viscous. No crystals.	Protein: <3 g/dL.
Glucose: <10 mg/dL.	WBC count: <200/mm^3. No abnormal cells/inclusions. Granulocytes <25%. RBC count: 0

Results for ANA, C3, uric acid, and RF for synovial fluid should be similar to results for serum.

Serous Fluid (Peritoneal/Pleural) Transudate and Exudate

Serous fluid is found in body cavities. Transudates result from impaired regulation of fluid balance, which causes fluid to leak from capillaries while exudates result from disorders of the surrounding membrane, such as cancer or infection, which allows larger molecules to leak through blood vessels.

Peritoneal /Pleural fluids	Transudate	Exudate
Appearance	Clear, watery	Cloudy
Sp. gravity	<1.015	>1.018
Protein	<2.5 g/dL	2.9 g/dL
Odor	None	Odor if infection present
Glucose	10-20 mg/dL	Very low
White blood cell count	<100 cells/mm^3	>1000 cells/mm^3
Red blood cell count	<1000 cells/mm^3	Varies
pH	7.60-7.64	<7.3
Pleural fluid to serum protein ratio	<0.5	>0.5
Pleural fluid to serum LDH ratio	<0.6	>0.6

Semen Analysis

Semen analysis is done to diagnose fertility problems. The sample of ejaculate should be transported at body temperature in a clean glass container for examination. A fresh sample at testing sight is preferable. A condom should not be used for collection. Semen is white/opaque and viscous with a distinctive musty odor. Composition:

- pH: 7.2-8.0
- Volume: 2-5 mL, <1.5 mL is abnormal.
- Clotting/Liquefaction: Usually complete in 15 to 20 minutes. Should complete within 30 minutes.
- Sperm count: >15 million/mL.
- Total sperm count: >39 million per ejaculation.
- Motility at 60 minutes: ≥40%.

- Vitality: ≥60%.
- Morphology: >25%-30% (preferably >70%) normal in appearance. Appearance: 50-70 μm in length with large oval head, slender tail (90% of length), and small neck.

Abnormalities that may require further testing include decreased sperm count and decreased motility. Sperm count decreased: hyperpyrexia, ejaculatory obstruction, orchitis, testicular failure/atrophy, varicocele, and post-vasectomy.

Sources of Error and Corrective Actions in Hematological Tests

Sources of **errors in hematological tests** include instrumentation errors (most common) and personal errors, most often associated with a failure to follow standard protocols:

1. Use of incorrect collection tube: Follow protocol and check requirements.
2. Hemolysis: Ensure proper collection, mixing, and storing of blood samples.
3. Incorrectly calibrated equipment: Follow manufacturer's guidelines and lab protocols.
4. Incorrectly prepared thin and thick blood films: Check film and redo if problems occur.
5. Dirty/defective equipment: Check all equipment before use.
6. Inaccurate use of equipment: Check directions for use if unsure or unfamiliar with equipment.
7. Improper technique: Follow established protocols every time.
8. Outdated reagent: Check dates and rotate supply.
9. Sample degraded: Process samples within prescribed time period.
10. Inaccurate cell counting: Make sure to be alert and exercise care.
11. Anticoagulant concentration too high: Adjust for high hematocrit levels.
12. Incorrect mixing of sample: Follow standard procedure, mix properly, avoiding excessive shaking.

Molecular Assays

Molecular assays, such as PCR-ELISA and fluorescence in situ hybridization, are able to detect molecules or specific sequences in the genetic code that are markers for specific disease processes. Assays may be qualitative or quantitative. Molecular assays, which require a blood or stool sample, are less invasive than biopsies. Tests utilize RNA or DNA to determine if there are abnormalities causing disease. Assays can be designed about specific drug targets or receptors and are important in development of drugs. A biochemical assay uses DNA to monitor chemical reactions. A functional assay measures a physiological response to a drug. During a molecular assay, nucleic acid is extracted and purified and then amplified to make multiple copies. Commercial molecular assays are approved by the FDA. CLIA establishes standards and requirements for laboratory-developed assays, which are often used for patient management. Molecular assays may be used to diagnose different types of malignancies, infections, genetic disorders, coagulation disorders, and HLA typing.

CBC and Differential Using Automated Hematology Instrumentation

Automated analyzers carry out the CBC and differential. Some analyzers are small and process one blood sample at a time. A sample is mixed and a small amount aspirated into the machine. Others are able to process dozens of samples, which are labeled and placed in special racks. Technology utilized in analyzers includes:

- Impedance analysis: Blood passes in a one-cell diameter stream through electrodes that pass a charge through the blood cells according to the cell size, allowing the analyzer to act as a cell counter able to count thousands of cells each second. The analyzer is able to differentiate and count RBCs, lymphocytes, and monocytes, but can only count total granulocytes, not differentiate them.

- Laser flow cytometry: Similar to impedance analysis except the stream passes through lasers, which measure absorbance, and are able to better differentiate cell morphology for the WBC differential.
- Fluorescent flow cytometry: Adds fluorescent reagents to show the ratio of nucleus to plasma for each cell in order to count platelets, reticulocytes, and nucleated RBCs.

Cytochemical Staining

Cytochemical staining is used to identify enzymes, cell type, or other substances in blood cell cytoplasm based on color reactions to a reagent. The purpose is to identify cells; diagnose, differentiate, and/or confirm diagnosis of leukemia; identify enzyme deficiencies; and detect abnormalities of cytoplasm. Cytochemical staining includes an enzyme plus a substrate (substance with which the enzyme will react) leading to an identifiable color change. Chemical stains may be enzymatic (myeloperoxidase, non-specific esterase, specific esterase, and tartrate-resistance acid phosphatase) or non-enzymatic (toluidine blue, PAS, Sudan black). The procedure will vary somewhat depending on the chemical stain utilized. Basic procedure:

- Fix a smear (air dried) with the appropriate fixative (such as cold buffered acetone or formalin vapors) for the prescribed period, ranging from seconds to 10-15 minutes.
- Process and stain the smear through various steps:
- Rinse with water or air wash for prescribed period of time.
- Incubate in substrate solution if required.
- Wash and stain as needed.
- Counterstain as needed.
- Rinse and air dry if needed.
- Note results and reaction product.

Peripheral Blood Smear and Bone Marrow Slides

Thin films for **blood smears and bone marrow smears** are the best choice for assessing the morphology of blood cells and verifying cell counts. Blood smears are often done when the results of the CBC were abnormal to check all 3 cells lines. Procedure:

- Transfer 4 mm diameter drop of EDTA-anticoagulated blood or bone marrow aspirant to end of one slide.
- Position a spreader slide at a 45° angle just ahead of the drop.
- Pull to spreader along the slide until it touches the drop.
- Allow the drop to spread along the spreader edge.
- Push the spreader to the other end of the slide, keeping the 45° angle, drawing the blood along the slide.
- Wave the slide to thoroughly dry blood.
- Stain (Wright or Wright-Giemsa) by flooding slide, drying for 3 minutes or more, and then rising with distilled/non-ionized water and air drying.

If streaks or lines are evident along the slide, the blood was clotting. Bone marrow smears are usually compared to a blood smear.

Identification of Malarial Parasites

Preparing slides and evaluating for **identification of malarial parasites** (*Plasmodium* spp.):

- Gather supplies: microscope, slides, slide spreaders, containers for Field stain, draining racks, applicator sticks.
- Obtain blood specimen (anticoagulated venous blood or non-anticoagulated capillary blood).

- Place one drop of blood on slide for a thin film to identify species and RBC morphology. Spread blood with spreader at ≤45° angle.
- Place 2-3 drops of blood on slide for thick film to detect density. Spread blood evenly over about a 1 cm area (should be translucent while wet).
- Label films and allow to dry for at least 30 minutes.
- Fix the thin film with methanol but not the thick. Stain thin film with Giemsa and thick with Field stain.
- Air dry.
- Examine under high-powered microscope and oil immersion.

Use thick film to determine density of parasites. *P. falciparum* has high density; *P. vivax,* medium, and *P. malariae,* low. Use thin film to identify the stages of the parasite (trophozoites, schizont, gametocyte). The RBCs are no longer visible but pink Schüffner's dots appear about parasites and trophozoite cytoplasm stains blue.

Use of Stains

Crystal violet can be used in the laboratory to determine the presence of Heinz bodies in red blood cells (erythrocytes). Prussian blue can be used to detect iron in bone marrow, peripheral blood, or in urine. Sudan black B is used to determine the presence of lipids (fats), and Wright's stain can be used to determine the presence of basophilic stippling. Howell-Jolly bodies, and Pappenheimer bodies.

MacConkey Agar

MacConkey agar is a medium used in the laboratory to grow mycobacteria, such as *Mycobacteria chelonae*, and to differentiate between different types of mycobacteria. It is also used to stain gram negative bacteria for lactose fermentation. MacConkey agar consists of lactose, peptone, bile salts, crystal violet dye, and a neutral red dye. The red dye is what stains the bacteria that are fermenting the lactose present in the agar. MacConkey agar is used to not only identify various fast-growing mycobacteria, but it can be used to identify other pathogens, such as *Salmonella* and *Shigella*.

Bacterial Culture Methods

Selective, Differential and Enrichment Media, Candle Jars, and Living Host Cells

A number of different **media** are utilized for bacterial cultures, which are used to increase the numbers of a microorganism, select specific types, or differentiate them:

1. Differential: The media changes in appearance with color change as a biochemical reaction to different bacteria, helping to distinguish different organisms.
2. Selective: The media encourages the growth of one type of microorganism while inhibiting the growth of others.
3. Enrichment: Media enriched with additives (such as sheep's blood) that encourages the growth of a specific type of microorganism.
4. Candle jar: Inoculated specimen plates are placed inside of a glass jar and a small candle placed on top of the upper plate. As the candle burns, it uses up most of the oxygen and the carbon dioxide stimulates anaerobic bacterial growth although some aerobic growth may also occur because of residual oxygen.
5. Living host cells: Used for some specific types of microorganisms that only grow in living cells, such as some leprosy.

Anaerobic Media and Techniques and Living Host Cells

Anaerobic microorganisms are most often found in abscesses and deep wounds, such as bites, blood, and cerebrospinal fluid. Aseptic technique is especially important to avoid contamination, and cotton swabs should not be used to collect a specimen because they may damage the microorganisms. Sample must be transported in an oxygen-free container.

- Anaerobic media: Pre-reduced anaerobically sterilized (PRAS) media is available, but is expensive and other media (selective, differential, or enriched) may be utilized as well if processed properly.
- Anaerobic techniques: Inoculated specimen plates are placed inside an anaerobic jar with an inlet and outlet and an electrified catalyst combines hydrogen and oxygen to provide anaerobic environment. With the gas pack, the inoculated plates are placed inside a container and water added combine hydrogen and oxygen, producing an anaerobic environment. Methylene blue is utilized as an anaerobic indicator.

Additives Used in Media Preparation

Media for culture must allow microorganisms to grow and reproduce, so various **additives** (nutrients or inhibitors) are added to an aqueous base to create different types of media. Complex media, which usually contain glucose and animal or plant proteins (protein hydrolysates such as tryptone), support various types of heterotrophic microorganisms. Defined media have exact percentages of various additives (such as mineral salts, growth factors, and simple carbohydrate) and support specific microorganisms and are generally required for microbiological assays. Selective media often have additives (such as mannitol) to suppress growth of undesirable microorganisms while promoting growth of others (such as *Staphylococcus aureus)*. Differential media have additives that help to distinguish different types of colonies. Enriched media contains additives (such as sheep blood or heated blood [chocolate]) to encourage increased growth of specific microorganisms. Commonly used additives include arginine, biotin, dextrin, galactose, glucose, lactose, mannitol, citric acid, sorbitol, and EDTA.

Mode of Action for Antimicrobial Agents

The mode of action of Gentamicin, Vancomycin, Clindamycin, Rifampin, Penicillin, and Tetracycline are explained below:

- Gentamicin works by interfering with protein synthesis. Gentamicin can be used to treat urinary tract infections.
- Vancomycin works by interfering with the synthesis of bacterial cell walls. Vancomycin can be used to treat serious respiratory infections in patients that are allergic to penicillins.
- Clindamycin works by interfering with protein synthesis. Clindamycin can be used to treat respiratory infections.
- Rifampin works by interfering with the synthesis of bacterial ribonucleic acid (RNA). Rifampin is used to treat tuberculosis.
- Penicillin works by interfering with the synthesis of bacterial cell walls. Penicillin can be used to treat pneumonia.
- Tetracycline works by interfering with the synthesis of bacterial RNA. It can be used to treat infections of the respiratory tract.

Culturing Clinical Specimens

Blood	Obtain two (anaerobic and aerobic) 8-10 mL specimens at temperature peak and/or multiple at 30-minute to 1-hour intervals and inoculate the blood culture vials. Incubate and monitor as per protocol. Gram stain samples from positive cultures and subculture for aerobic (sheep blood, chocolate agar) and anaerobic organisms according to protocol (usually after 18-48 hours). Incubate at 35°-37°C for up to 7 days and inspect at least 2 times daily.
Urine	Obtain clean catch or catheterized specimen in sterile container. Process immediately or store specimen at 4°C. Prepare a slide for gram staining with one drop of mixed (not centrifuged) urine and examine under microscope or conduct the leukocyte esterase strip test. Negative findings generally indicate culture is unnecessary, but positive findings should be followed by inoculation of a MacConkey agar plate with incubation at 35°-37°C for 24-48 hours.
Stool	Collect specimen prior to beginning antibiotics in a sterile container or use cotton-tipped swab inserted into the rectum and rotated to obtain a fecal sample. Insert swab into sterile tube. The specimen should be processed as soon as possible or stored at 4°C. Specimen should be examined microscopically and plates inoculated. A fecal suspension with saline may be necessary for swabs or solid stool specimens if multiple plates must be inoculated. This also helps eliminate organic matter. Various types of agar may be used depending on the suspected organisms. Incubate at 35°-37°C for 24-48 hours.
Sputum	Collect sputum specimen in wide-mouthed sterile container and process within one hour. Record macroscopic appearance and prepare a gram-stain for microscopic examination. If fewer than 10 PMNs are noted per epithelial cells, the specimen should be rejected. If more, agar plates (various types) should be inoculated and incubated 35°-37°C for 24-48 hours (inspect after 18 hours).
Throat (upper respiratory)	Collect 2 specimens with sterile swabs rubbed over the back of the throat and tonsillar areas, avoiding the tongue and other structures, and place in sterile tube for transfer. Process within 4 hours or place in transport medium. Gram-staining is generally done only on specific request. Inoculate a blood agar (low glucose) by rubbing the swab over 1 quadrant and streak the remaining quadrants with a sterile loop. Place a bacitracin disk and a co-trimoxazole disk over the streaked area to aid in identification of bacteria. Incubate at 35°-37°C for 18 hours and inspect for colonies and then inspect again at 48 hours. Gram-stain colony samples to aid in identification.
Cerebrospinal fluid	Collect 5 to 10 mL CSF in 2 sterile tubes and process immediately. The CSF should be assessed macroscopically and microscopically through direct microscopy, gram-stain, and acid-fast stain. Inoculate plates appropriate to bacteria identified through microscopy or multiple media if unclear and incubate for at least 3 days with temperature and conditions determined by the type of agar and environment required for suspected organisms (aerobic, anaerobic).
Wound	Collect specimen through aspiration (preferred) of exudate or tissue sample or by wiping the wound with 2 cotton swabs and placing swabs in sterile container, in transport medium if processing cannot be done immediately. The exudate should be examined with direct, Gram-stain, and acid-fast stain microscopy and macroscopically (color, consistency, odor). Depending on results of the microscopic examination, various types of plates (minimum 3) should be inoculated. If using a swab for inoculation, wipe the swab across one quadrant of a plate and streak the remaining quadrants with a wire loop. Incubation time, temperature, and environment depend on the type of plate and the suspected organisms.

Abscess	Similar to wound culture although aspirant only is generally used. Organisms may be polymicrobial, including both aerobic and anaerobic bacteria, depending on the site of the abscess. Culturing for anaerobic bacteria (both gram-negative and gram-positive) should always be included, so the specimen must be protected from exposure to oxygen and incubation done at 35°C for 48 hours and then examined.
Genital fluids	Females: Collect specimen with pelvic examination and speculum moistened only with water. Wipe away mucus about the cervix with a cotton swab/ball and discard. Then insert a cotton swab and wipe the vaginal posterior fornix for the first sample, use another swab to collect an endocervical sample by inserting the swab into the cervix and rotating it for 10 seconds. Males: Collect oropharyngeal, urethral, anorectal specimens in a similar manner, inserting swab 3 to 4 cm inside urethra and 4 to 5 cm inside anus/rectum. Examination: Examine macroscopically for color and odor and through direct and gram-stain microscopy. Culturing should be done to identify *Neisseria gonorrhoeae* (especially in females) with direct inoculation of Thayer-Martin agar incubated at 35°C in candle-jar environment for 48 hours (checked daily for colonies).
Ear exudates	Collect specimens with two swabs inserted gently into the ear canal and rotated. Examine through direct and Gram-stain microscopy. Culture is usually carried out on MacConkey medium, blood agar, and Sabouraud dextrose medium with antibiotics, depending on the type of bacteria observed through microscopy with temperature and environment also dependent on suspected bacteria.
Eye exudate	Collect 2 specimens with a sterile cotton swab from the lower conjunctival sac and from the inner canthus of each eye and place in sterile tubes. Examine (first swabs) through direct, Gram-stain, and Giemsa stain microscopically and then carry out cultures (second swabs). Volume of bacteria for both ear and eye exudates tends to be low, so antibiotic disks are generally not used. Media commonly used includes MacConkey agar (under aerobic condition), blood agar (candle jar), and chocolate agar (candle jar). Incubate 18-24 hours, examine, and incubate another 48 hours if necessary.
Tissue	Collect specimens through surgical procedure or endoscopy and place in sterile container in transport medium. Examine macroscopically and microscopically. Process the tissue sample as per protocol for type of tissue and inoculate various types of culture media, depending on the tissue type and suspected microorganisms. Incubate at 35 to 37°C for times indicated for media.
IV catheter tips	Collect the IV catheter intact and transport in sterile container. Cut a 5 cm section from the catheter tip and roll that four times over a solid medium plate or immerse the section in broth culture medium. Incubate at 35° to 37°C for the times indicated for media and examine for colonies (>15 significant). Various other methods may be utilized, and blood cultures are usually done simultaneously.
IUD	Similar to procedures for IV catheter tips. Endocervical (and sometimes blood) cultures are usually done simultaneously.

Processing and Planting of Specimens

Obtaining Inoculum from Agar and Broth

Processing and planting of specimens: Media used for cultures must be sterilized and maintained in sterile conditions and organisms transferred to the media using aseptic transfer techniques. Tube caps are removed and tops heated (up draft) to keep contamination away from the inside. Inoculation is typically made with a sterile inoculating needle (agar deeps) or wire loop (agar plates/broths). The inoculating needle or wire loop must be heated to red hot and cooled before transfer. To obtain inoculum:

- Agar plate: Lift one side of the lid (do not completely uncover) and use the wire loop to lift one colony (or part of a large colony) of the surface.
- Agar slant: Use the wire loop to scrape inoculum from the surface.
- Broth: Mix by shaking slightly and then immerse the loop and withdraw carefully (a film should be noted across the loop).

Note: For agar deep, obtain inoculum with a sterile needle.

Inoculating Agar and Broth

Always maintain aseptic technique. To inoculate:

- Agar deep: Insert the needle straight to the bottom and withdraw straight.
- Agar plate: Lift one side of the lid and slide the loop in horizontally, streaking the inoculum back and forth on the surface only. Reflame the loop after each third of the plate is streaked, reinoculate, turn the plate 90° and continue until the entire plate (or 3 quadrants) is streaked. Invert plate for incubation.
- Agar slant: Either insert loop to the bottom of the tube and withdraw straight (for growth pattern) or in back-and-forth manner (for increased growth).
- Broth: Swish the loop back and forth about the tube.

Once inoculation is complete, then the plate/tube is placed in the incubator with the temperature and duration determined by the type of medium and the type of organism.

Staining of Flagella

The most common technique used in the laboratory for the staining of flagella is the Leifson staining technique. Tannic acid-base fuchsin solution is used to stain the flagella that make bacteria mobile. The stain precipitates out along the filaments of the flagella, and the diameter of the flagella is increased. This then allows for the flagella to be easily visualized using light microscopy. The technique needs to be performed with care, however, to achieve accurate results Various aspects of the test need to be checked, such as the cleanliness of the glass slides used, the pH of the stain used, and the actual time the specimen spends submerged in stain.

Agar Diffusion Testing

Agar diffusion testing determines the antimicrobial effectiveness of a chemical. Streak a bacteria sample onto a nutrient-rich agar plate. The bacteria must be uniformly distributed on the plate, and Mueller-Hinton agar is the preferred agar for this analysis. Pipette various chemicals that are being tested onto numbered paper disks. Place these paper disks onto the streaked agar plate. Incubate at 37°C. Chemicals leach from the paper disks and spread outward onto the agar plate. Bacterial growth is not as prevalent in a clear ring surrounding a paper disk, so the chemical on that disk has antimicrobial effectiveness. Measure the clear areas (zones of inhibition) and compare the ring size to a standard atlas of zones of inhibition. The widest ring shows the most effective chemical.

Dilution Test

The tube dilution test determines if chemicals being tested are either bactericidal or bacteriostatic in nature. Chemicals that are bactericidal are those that kill bacteria, while chemicals that are bacteriostatic do not kill bacteria, rather they inhibit the growth and reproduction of bacteria. Place a bacteria specimen in a tube, along with the particular chemical that is being tested. Place this mixture onto a nutrient-rich agar plate. If the bacteria are able to grow on the plate at all, then the chemical that is being tested is likely to have some bacteriostatic properties, since the bacteria were not killed.

However, if no bacteria grow on the nutrient-rich agar plate, the bacteria must have been killed by the chemical being tested, which would make that chemical bactericidal.

Testing for Multi-Drug-Resistant Tuberculosis

Testing for **multi-drug-resistant tuberculosis** (*Mycobacterium tuberculosis*) includes:

- Agar proportion: Use Felsin quadrant plates, which contain an antibiotic-impregnated disk in 3 quadrants with the remaining quadrant serving as the control. Molten Middlebrook 7H11 agar medium is poured over the antimicrobial disks and incubated overnight to allow the antibiotic agent to diffuse through the medium. Then each quarter is inoculated and the plate sealed and incubated at 37° C for 3 to 4 weeks. The organism is susceptible to the antibiotic if there is >200 colonies in the control quadrant and none in the antibiotic-containing quadrant.
- 96 well microtiter plate (MYCOTB): This method requires first growing colonies of the microorganism and then inoculating the wells in the microtiter plate. The plate contains 12 antimicrobial drugs in different concentrations (isoniazid, rifampin, ethambutol, kanamycin, cycloserine, amikacin, moxifloxacin, ofloxacin, rifabutin, streptomycin, ethionamide, and para-aminosalicylic acid. (Note pyrazinamide must be tested for separately because it requires an acidic environment). The plate is incubated for 14 days and the growth in each well is evaluated utilizing a mirror box or an semi-automatic plate reader.

Oxidase Test

The oxidase test is used to distinguish bacteria on the basis of whether they contain cytochrome c oxidase by using disks that contain a reagent that changes color when oxidized. Moisten each disk containing the reagent with de-ionized water. Place a sample of the bacteria on each disk with the reagent. After three minutes, observe the color of the disks. If there has been a color change to either maroon, blue, or black, then the reagent has been oxidized, and the bacteria is oxidase positive, or OX+. Oxidase positive bacteria can use oxygen for energy production, and they do contain cytochrome c oxidase. The Pseudomonadaceae are oxidase positive. If there is no color change after three minutes, then the reagent is reduced and the bacteria are oxidase negative (OX-). The Enterobacteriaceae are oxidase negative.

Nagler Test

The Nagler test is used to identify bacterial organisms that can produce lecithinases (phospholipases). One example of such an organism is *Clostridium perfringens*. Place the sample in question on an agar medium containing egg yolk. On one half of the agar medium, add the antitoxin for *Clostridium perfringens* type A. After incubation, a positive Nagler test will show the half of the test plate that contains the antitoxin is clear and has no evidence of lecithinase production. The half of the test plate that did not contain the antitoxin will show evidence of the production of lecithinase as an opaque area surrounding the bacterial sample.

Niacin Test

The niacin test is used to identify the presence of a specific type of mycobacteria, *Mycobacterium tuberculosis*. This particular mycobacterium releases a large quantity of niacin (B_3) during its metabolic processes. All mycobacteria release a certain amount of niacin, but only Mycobacterium tuberculosis releases enough to be of use in the niacin test. Culture the sample on egg based media for a three to four week incubation period before niacin testing. Add a cyanogen bromide (CNBr) solution and an aniline solution to the egg based bacterial culture. If niacin is present, a color change to yellow will be seen. If there is no color change, then *Mycobacterium tuberculosis* is not present. Care should be taken when performing the niacin test because cyanogen bromide solution is highly toxic. Wear a respirator, gloves, and use a fume hood.

Indole Test

The indole test is performed on bacteria to determine its ability to produce indole from the degradation of tryptophan. Incubate a bacterial culture in a peptone or tryptophan broth for a 24 to 48 hour period. After this incubation period, add Kovac's reagent or Ehrlich's reagent to the broth and bacterial culture mixture. If the surface layer of the broth changes to red-violet or red in color, then the test is positive. An example of a bacterium that will have a positive result is *E. coli*. If the surface layer is yellow, however, the test is negative. *Salmonella* results in a negative indole test. A third result is possible, and that is if the surface layer of the broth turns orange. This is called a variable result. The variable result is due to presence of methyl indole, instead of indole.

Streptococcal Testing

Throat Swabs and Cultures for Beta-Hemolysis Screening

***Streptococcus* infections include strep throat, scarlet fever, rheumatic fever, necrotizing fasciitis, urinary tract infections, psoriasis, and pneumonia.**	
Throat swabs: rapid enzyme immunoassay (more accurate for positives than negatives) (group A)	A number of different rapid strep kits are available that are able to detect strep group A. The tests usually begin with a tonsillar and throat swab. The swab is then swirled inside of a tube holding a mixture of 2 reagents, left in place for about 1 minute, and then removed and a test strip inserted, timed, and checked against a color chart. Antibody/antigen sensitivity tests also help to identify strep.
Beta-hemolytic strep (group B) screening for *S. agalactiae*.	Commonly colonizes in intestinal, urinary, and reproductive systems and can infect the fetus in late pregnancy, so screening of pregnant women is done routinely with rectal and vaginal cultures because most are asymptomatic. While the strep is not usually pathogenic to the mother, the newborn may develop pneumonia (newborns lack alveolar macrophages) or meningitis.

Bacterial Identification

Bacterial identification	• Streptococci are gram-positive cocci that occur in pairs or chains and are facultative anaerobes. Streptococci grow on blood agar, chocolate agar, and (some species) on PEA. Cultured colonies are small, gray, and slightly raised and appear translucent with a margin around the entire colony. • Streptococci are catalase negative, esculin negative, MSA, and optochin negative, and these tests can differentiate strep from other cocci. • Alpha-hemolytic strep (*S. pneumoniae*, which is optochin susceptible and bile soluble) exhibits only partial hemolysis. • Beta-hemolytic strep includes group A strep (*S. pyogenes*, which exhibit strong beta-hemolysis and bacitracin inhibition) and group B strep (*S. agalactiae*, identified by the CAMP test). Beta-hemolytic strep cases complete hemolysis.

Gram's Method of Staining Bacteria

Gram staining method is used to distinguish between gram-positive and gram-negative bacteria in the laboratory. Stain the sample with crystal violet. Next, treat the sample with a solution of iodine. Add alcohol or another organic solvent to the sample. Examine the sample under the microscope. Gram-positive bacteria will still be stained a violet/blue color. Gram-negative bacteria, however, will be colorless. In order to make the gram-negative bacteria stand out, counterstain the sample with safrinin. This counterstain will make the gram-negative bacteria appear red in color, and the gram-positive bacteria will still appear violet/blue in color.

USE OF STAINS

Below are examples of how crystal violet, Wright's stain, Sudan black B, and Giemsa can be used in the laboratory:

- Crystal violet is used for the gram staining of bacterial cell walls. Gram-negative bacteria will appear red or pink in color, and gram-positive bacteria will appear dark blue or violet in color when treated with crystal violet.
- Wright's stain is used to help distinguish blood cells. It can be used with either blood or bone marrow samples. Often it is used when performing white blood cell (WBC) counts if infections are expected in the patient.
- Sudan black B is a stain that is used to identify the presence of triglycerides or lipids. Sudan black B will stain these compounds a bluish-black color.
- Giemsa stain is a stain that can be used to identify bacteria and other parasites. Giemsa stain can be used with blood films, blood smears, or bone marrow samples. Giemsa stain will stain parasites or bacterial cells a purple color, while the human cells will be colored pink. Giemsa stain is made of a combination of eosin and methylene blue.

IMMUNOLOGY

Immunology involves the immune response to foreign substances (microorganisms and proteins), which provides defense (attacks antigens/pathogens), homeostasis (digests damaged cellular materials), and surveillance (destroys mutated forms). All cells carry antigens, which are composed of proteins. The body usually recognizes its own antigens and does not attack them (except in autoimmune disorders). B-lymphocytes (produced in bone marrow) produce antigen-binding proteins (immunoglobulins) on their cell membranes. When the Ig binds with an antigen, this stimulates the B-cell to produce plasma cells, which in turn produce further immunoglobulins that are released as antibodies: IgM (first released), IgG (second released and more specific to an antigen), IgA (present in secretions) and IgE (triggers basophils and mast cells to release histamine). T-lymphocyte helper cells (CD4 cells) (produced in the thymus gland) secrete cytokines (hormones that signal other cells) when they contact foreign antigens. T-lymphocyte cytotoxic cells (CD8 cells) directly destroy foreign antigens that are outside of infected cells (not adhered).

FACTORS AFFECTING ANTIGEN-ANTIBODY REACTIONS

Factors affecting antigen-antibody reactions include:

- Temperature: Antigen-antibody reactions are usually more stable at low temperatures, and the strength of bonds tends to increase as the temperature rises.
- pH: Equilibrium constant is attained at 6.5-8.4. Extremes alter the antibody molecule.
- Incubation time: Duration needed to reach equilibrium varies according to the ionic strength: faster at low strength and slower at high strength. Duration should be at least 20 minutes at low strength.
- Ionic strength: Reactions vary in time needed to reach equilibrium depending on the concentration of ions. At low strength, gamma globulins aggregate, resulting in increased complement fraction attachment and RBV aggregation.
- Antibody/antigen excess: Numbers of antigens or antibodies are so high that antigen-antibody crosslinking (agglutination) is reduced because of the excess of either antigens or antibodies.
- Enhancement media: Reaction may vary depending on the type of enhancement media utilized.
- Blood-banking technology: Rare blood types may cause unexpected reactions.
- Dilution/Concentration: Can alter the number of immunoglobulins by increasing or decreasing dissociation.

Direct Coombs Test

The direct Coombs test is used to determine if complement system factors or antibodies are bound to antigens found on the surface of red blood cells in a test sample. In this test, a patient's test sample is washed, which removes the serum from the red blood cells. The red blood cells are then added to the Coombs reagent. The Coombs reagent is an antihuman globulin. The antihuman globulin will cause the red blood cells in the test sample to clot (agglutinate) if those red blood cells have antibodies or complement system factors attached to their surfaces. This result is indicative of a positive direct Coombs test. If the agglutination does not occur, then the direct Coombs test is negative. The direct Coombs test is used most often if hemolytic anemia (immune controlled) is suspected. In patients whose red blood cells are being hemolyzed by their immune system, a positive Coombs test will occur.

Indirect Coombs Test

The indirect Coombs test is performed in vitro to understand and determine the presence of reactions between antibodies and antigens in a red blood cell sample. In the laboratory, red blood cells are washed and then added to a test serum. If the test serum contains red blood cells that have antigens or antibodies attached to their surfaces, the antibodies will bind onto the surfaces of the washed red blood cells. Next, the red blood cells are then washed several more times with a saline solution, and then added to the Coombs reagent (an antihuman globulin). If antibodies attached to the washed red blood cells previously, the red blood cells will clot (agglutinate) when the Coombs reagent is added. If the agglutination occurs, the indirect Coombs test positive. The indirect Coombs test can be used for: Antibody identification, determining antibody concentrations in serum or plasma before blood transfusion, titrations, or determining red blood cell phenotypes.

Kleihauer-Betke Test

The Kleihauer-Betke test is an acid elution test used to determine the severity or presence of fetal-maternal hemorrhage postpartum. This is accomplished by determining the quantity of fetal red blood cells or hemoglobin present in the mother's blood stream after delivery. This test is performed when a Rh negative mother has given birth. In this particular test, at a pH of 3.2, a sample of maternal blood is stained with erythrosine B-hematoxylin. Once the stain is applied, the adult hemoglobin (which is soluble in the acid solution) will turn pale. Sometimes the adult hemoglobin is said to become ghost-like. The fetal hemoglobin, on the other end, is not soluble in the acid solution, and remains bright pink. Depending on the amount of fetal hemoglobin present in the maternal blood sample, the appropriate dosage of Rh immune globulin (RhIg) can be administered to the mother to help prevent the formation of Rh antibodies in the mother's blood.

Weil-Felix Test

The Weil-Felix test is used to define the presence of *Rickettsia*, bacteria that are often carried by lice, ticks, and fleas. Populations of *Rickettsia* that are present in an affected patient's blood serum cause the production of various antibodies. These antibodies have the ability to react with other types of bacteria. In the Weil-Felix test, another type of bacteria (often *Proteus vulgaris*) is added to a patient's blood serum. This bacteria serves as an antigen and will react (agglutinate) with the antibodies produced from the *Rickettsia* in the patient's blood serum. This agglutination can help identify which type of *Rickettsia* afflicts the patient. Some rickettsial diseases that can be identified by this method are Rocky Mountain spotted fever, trench fever, typhus, and scrub typhus.

ELISA Test

ELISA stands for enzyme-linked immunosorbent assay, an immunoassay test that identifies the presence of specific substances, like the AIDS virus. ELISA can identify hormones, proteins, antibodies, or antigens. Add an antibody specific to the substance of interest to the test system. Mix a sample of the pure substance in question with an enzyme. This creates an enzyme-linked substance. Add both the enzyme-linked substance and the blood serum to the test system. If the serum contains the substance of interest, less of the enzyme-linked substance will be able to bind to the antibody that was added. If there is no substance of interest in the serum, more enzyme-linked substance will be able to bond to the available antibody. Finally, add the particular substance that the enzyme acts on to the system. Measure the product produced via a color analysis. This test is very sensitive and is used frequently to confirm a less sensitive, but cheaper, screening test.

MHA-TP

The **microhemagglutination test for *Treponema pallidum* (MHA-TP),** a gram-negative spirochete, is a nontreponemal antibody tests that assesses serum for antibodies to syphilis although this particular test has been generally replaced by other tests that are more specific, such as fluorescent treponemal antibody absorption (FTA-ABS), immunoassays, and molecular testing. MHA-TP can be used to confirm a positive diagnosis of syphilis on other tests. MHA-TP is able to detect antibodies to *T. pallidum* and is used for all stages of syphilis except during the first month of infection. One of the problems with MHA-TP is that false positives may occur in the presence of other infections, so it is not specific to syphilis: mononucleosis, Lyme disease, malaria, relapsing fever, leptospirosis, and leprosy. Patients with systemic lupus erythematosus may also have a false-positive on the test.

Febrile Agglutination Tests

Febrile agglutinins are antibodies that are active at normal body temperature and can cause their antigens (such as RBCs, proteins) to clump when exposed to each other, resulting in a fever. Febrile agglutinins are present in some disorders, such as systemic lupus erythematosus, hemolytic anemia, inflammatory bowel disease, and lymphoma. They may also occur in response to some infections (salmonella, brucellosis, typhoid fever) and when taking some medications (penicillin, methyldopa), so these medications may interfere with test results. To identify an infection, a blood sample is taken when a patient is actively infected (with fever and symptoms) or during convalescence, diluted (20-40 times), and mixed with antigens of a specific infectious microorganism. This sample is then examined to determine if an antigen-antibody reaction has occurred. Increased IgM usually indicates a new infection and increased IgG indicates a chronic infection or history of infection.

CRP Agglutination Slide Tests and ASO

C-reactive protein (CRP) agglutination slide tests can be used to screen patients for CRP (qualitative test) or to determine the titer (quantitative test). A number of different test kits are available, so procedures may vary.

Qualitative test	Quantitative test
Add latex solution to positive and negative controls and serum (or diluted and undiluted serum), mix, and agitate for 2 minutes to observe for agglutination (clumping) in serum, a reaction indicating the presence of C-reactive protein.	Mix serum samples to different dilutions in saline and conduct test similar to qualitative method to determine the highest dilution that shows agglutination (positive reaction).

Antistreptolysin O screen and titer (ASO) identifies the presence of streptolysin O antibodies, which form in response to the streptolysin O enzyme (antigen) secreted by group A β-hemolytic streptococci. The antibodies are present within one week and peak at 2-3 weeks after onset of streptococcal infection. Increased titer is present with strep-associated rheumatic fever, scarlet fever, endocarditis, and glomerulonephritis.

Rheumatoid Arthritis (RA) Tests

Rheumatoid factor (RF)	Normal value 0-20 IU/mL. Assesses for macroglobulin type antibody that is present in connective tissue disease. Non-specific for RA
Anti-citrullinated protein antibody (ACPA):	Normal values: • Negative: <20. • Weakly positive: 20-39. • Moderately positive: 40-59. • Strongly positive: >60. Assesses for autoantibodies against citrullinated proteins, to which those with RA react.
Erythrocyte sedimentation rate (ESR):	Normal values: • Age <50: 0-15 mm/h males and 0-25 mm/h females. • Age >50: 0-20 mm/h males and 0-30 mm/h females. Inflammation causes increased globulins or fibrinogens, and these cause RBCs to clump and fall to the bottom of a vertical test tube. ESR is nonspecific for RA, but increased ESR may indicate increased inflammation.
C-reactive protein (CRP):	Normal value <1 mg/dL. Assesses for abnormal glycoproteins, which are produced by the liver when inflammation is present. CRP is non-specific for RA.

SLE Tests

Systemic lupus erythematosus (SLE) is a chronic connective tissue disorder believed triggered by an antibody-antigen immune response to an environmental agent, resulting in widespread damage of vessels and organs, primarily in females. SLE ranges from mild to widely disseminated, and may include arthralgia, "butterfly" rash, arthritis, anemia, leukopenia, visceral lesions, CNS involvement (seizures, headaches, psychosis), fever, and lymphadenopathy. There is no single specific test for SLE, but rather diagnosis is based on the results of a number of imaging studies (x-rays, ECG) and laboratory studies:

- Complete blood cell count (CDC): May show anemia with erythrocytopenia and/or leukopenia.
- Erythrocyte sedimentation rate (ESR): Rate increases with SLE.
- Renal and hepatic function tests: Abnormalities may indicate lesions in the kidneys or liver.
- Urinalysis: Protein may be in the urine with renal lesions.
- Antinuclear antibody test: Presence of antibodies indicates an immune response. While results are not specific to ANA, this test is used primarily as part of SLE diagnosis.
- Renal biopsy: To determine type and degree of kidney involvement.

ANA Tests

ANA is used to diagnose autoimmune disorders, primarily SLE, Sjögren syndrome, scleroderma, and rheumatic diseases, which involve multiple body systems. Diagnosis depends on the ANA pattern exhibited and associated antibodies. Laboratories vary in reference ranges. Antinuclear antibodies are autoimmune antibodies that mistakenly target native tissue and cells as foreign. ANA is often done in conjunction with other autoantibody tests, such as anti-DNA and anti-nucleolar.

Results	Testing
Positive or negative: ANA results vary depending on the specific test used and the lab.	Collect serum (3 mL) in red-capped tube for indirect fluorescent antibody (IFA) or immunoassay. Immunoassay is less sensitive that IFA, so initial screening may be done by immunoassay with confirmation testing by IFA.

Antigen Detection

Antigen detection for specific organisms is frequently done as part of diagnostic studies. Various tests can be used. Enzyme immunoassays (EIA/ELISA) use various techniques, depending on the target antigen and microorganism. Techniques include binding an antibody (specific to the antigen under study) to a micro-dilution tray and adding the antigen, incubating, and washing it. Then, a second enzyme-labeled antibody is utilized to detect the antigen through a color change. With use of the immunochromatographic membrane, an antigen is absorbed through a nitrocellulose membrane and the color change occurs on the membrane when reagents are added. Latex agglutination tests, in which the antigen is affixed to latex beads, are used to identify carbohydrate antigens that occur on encapsulated organisms. With the Western blot test, antigens are put on a nitrocellulose strip and incubated with the antibody specimen and treated with an enzyme-labeled antibody and color change observed. Western blot is used frequently to confirm diagnosis of HIV.

Pregnancy Tests

Human chorionic gonadotropin (hCG) (quantitative)	Negative: <5 mIU/mL 2 weeks: 5-100 mIU/mL 4 weeks: 10,000-80,000 mIU/mL 5-12 weeks: 90,000-500,000 mIU/mL 13-24 weeks: 5000-80,000 mIU/mL 26-28 weeks: 3000-15,000 mIU/mL	Measures the amount of hCG in the blood. Obtain 1 mL sample in red or tiger-capped tube or 1 mL in heparinized green-capped tube for immunoassay.
hCG (qualitative)	Negative if absent Positive if present	Measures only presence or absence of hCG and cannot determine weeks of gestation. Obtain 1 mL sample in red or tiger-capped tube or 1 mL in heparinized green-capped tube.
hCG urine (home-pregnancy test)	Positive or negative	A test strip of some type is used and color change noted.

Viral/Retroviral Laboratory Tests

Cytomegalovirus	Negative: ≤0.9 index Indeterm: 0.91-1.09 Positive: ≥1.1 index	Obtain 1 mL sample in red-capped tube for enzyme immunoassay for antibody detection.
Retrovirus	Negative: 0 present	Obtain 1 mL sample in red or tiger-capped tube for enzyme immunoassay for antibody detection. Tests may include ELISA, nucleic acid testing, PCR, western blot.
Epstein-Barr	Negative <17 u/mL Indeterm 18.0-21.9 u/mL Positive >22 u/mL	Obtain 1 mL sample in gold-capped serum separator tube for chemiluminescent immunoassay.
Rubella	Negative: ≤0.9 index Indeterm: 0.91-1.09 Positive: ≥1.1 index	Obtain 1 mL sample in red-capped tube for chemiluminescent immunoassay.

HIV Tests

These tests screen for the presence of antibodies and/or antigens to HIV. The antigen is present before antibodies, so tests that include antigen assessment can give earlier results.

Rapid HIV test	Negative or positive	Most test only for antibodies, but newer tests may test for antigens as well. Tests can be done on blood, plasma, or oral fluid, but the rapid test is most often done with an oral swab with results (usually color change) available within seconds to minutes, depending on the test. These tests are less accurate than other tests, so findings must be confirmed.
HIV-1/HIV-2 test (serum)	Negative or positive	Screens for HIV antigen (p24) and HIV-1 and HIV-2 antibodies. Obtain 1 mL sample in red-capped tube for enzyme immunoassay. Confirmatory tests required.
IFA/Western blot	Negative or positive	Done for confirmatory testing when initial screening tests are positive or with individuals at high risk with negative screening tests.

Fecal Occult Blood and Immunochemical Tests

Stool may be examined macroscopically for volume, odor, color, consistency, mucus, and microscopically to identify the presence of cells (leukocytes, epithelial cells) and other materials (meat fibers). **Tests for occult blood** commonly include:

- **Fecal occult blood test (FOBT):** This test detects blood that has occurred from anywhere in the digestive tract because the blood reacts to the guaiac the test card is coated with. This test cannot distinguish between bleeding from the upper GI tract and the lower GI tract, so it is less specific than the FIT.
- **Fecal immunochemical test (FIT):** This test detects blood in the stool from lower GI bleeding through the use of antibodies against human hemoglobin (so it does not react to animal hemoglobin from ingested meats). FIT does not detect upper GI bleeding because the hemoglobin has been broken down by the digestive process by the time it reaches the rectum and is expelled.

MRSA

Methicillin-resistant *Staphylococcus aureus* (MRSA) was first identified in 1961 in Europe after the development and overuse of synthetic penicillins caused *Staphylococcus aureus* to mutate into resistant strains. Since 1961, MRSA has infected millions of people worldwide. MRSA is resistant to methicillin and other β-lactam antibiotics, such as amoxicillin and oxacillin, and sometimes other classes of antibiotics. *Staphylococcus* is able to form biofilms, which aids in resistance. Healthcare-associated MRSA infections most commonly involve surgical sites, urinary tract, blood stream, and lungs (pneumonia). Because of increased awareness and better practices, MRSA HAIs decreased by 54% between 2004 and 2011 but still pose a threat to patients because of the severity of some infections and the risk of resistance to other drugs. Community-acquired MRSA most commonly results in skin infections, such as folliculitis, and can easily spread to others where groups of people are in close contact, such as in day cares, gyms, schools, and barracks.

MDRO and Vancomycin-Resistant *Enterococcus*

Multi-Drug-Resistant Organisms (MDRO)

MDROs are those that have mutated and developed forms that are resistant to multiple antibiotics. Initially, resistance developed to one class of antibiotics, such as β-lactams, which resulted in methicillin-resistant *Staphylococcus aureus* infections and penicillin-resistant *Streptococcus pneumoniae,* but bacteria continued to mutate, becoming resistant to more classes of antibiotics and severely limiting the antibiotic arsenal needed for treatment. Of current concern is extended-spectrum beta-lactamases (ESBLs), resistant to cephalosporins and monobactams; and multi-drug-resistant tuberculosis (MDR).

Vancomycin-Resistant Enterococcus (VRE)

Up until the 1980s, most enterococci responded to vancomycin, a strong antibiotic, but the increased use of antibiotics for all types of infection resulted in mutations that rendered some enterococci species vancomycin-resistant (VRE), leaving few options for treatment of severe infection. There are currently 6 different forms (A-G) of vancomycin resistance. For example, the Van-A form is resistant to vancomycin and teicoplanin (an alternative antibiotic for severe infections).

String Test

The string test, sometimes referred to as the Entero-test, is used to help determine the presence of a parasitic infection. Usually, stool samples are examined first for parasites. If no parasites are found and the patient is still symptomatic, the string test is employed. Attach a string to a weighted gelatin capsule and observe the patient as he/she swallows it. Approximately four hours later, retrieve the string through the patient's mouth. Examine any mucus from the intestines that is attached to the string under a microscope. Any parasites and/or eggs that are present can then be seen. This test is not very common, but it can help determine the presence of various parasites, such as *Giardia lamblia*, a common cause of gastrointestinal disease.

Enterobiasis Tape Test

The enterobiasis tape test is used to discover pinworms (enterobiasis). Use a flashlight and sticky tape to gather pinworms and pinworm eggs from the patient's anus as he/she sleeps. If the patient wishes to do it, it must be done first thing in the morning because pinworms tend to deposit eggs near the anus overnight, and disappear back into the rectum. Touch the sticky side of the tape onto a clean glass slide, and examine it under the microscope. Any pinworms or pinworm eggs that are present will be seen at low magnification. Sometimes, more than one enterobiasis tape test needs to be done to achieve accurate results. Performing the test for three days straight is sufficient. If pinworms or their eggs are found, the infection is usually treated with the Mebendazole.

KOH Test

The KOH (potassium hydroxide) test is the first that should be used to identify fungi in a sample of human skin, nails, tissue, or hair. The KOH test dissolves the human cells, leaving only the fungal cells for examination. Scrape a sample of human cells suspected to contain a fungus onto a laboratory slide. Add several drops of 10% KOH in water to the slide. Cover the slide with a coverslip. Warm the slide in a Bunsen burner flame, but do not boil it. Examine it under a microscope. The KOH will have dissolved the human cells. Any visible cells are fungal. The differences in the composition of the cell walls of human and fungal cells allow for this reaction with the KOH solution.

Western Blot Test

The Western blot test is used in the laboratory to help confirm or deny the presence of HIV virus. Unlike the Southern blot and Northern blot tests, this test can test for both DNA and RNA protein fragments. Gel electrophoresis is used to separate these fragments of the viruses' DNA and RNA, and then they are covered with a membrane composed of nitrocellulose. The patient's serum is reacted with these separated DNA and RNA fragments. If the patient's serum contains antibodies for the HIV virus, those antibodies will bind to the DNA and RNA fragments present. This binding will produce a characteristic pattern (referred to as the characteristic blot), which can then be visualized. This pattern can then confirm the presence of the HIV virus in the patient's blood serum.

Southern Blot Test and Northern Blot Test

The Southern blot test is used to identify DNA (deoxyribonucleic acid) fragments in the laboratory. In this test, gel electrophoresis is used to separate fragments of DNA. Then, these fragments are covered with a membrane consisting of nitrocellulose. Finally, a specific probe is used to identify the fragments of DNA. The Northern blot test is used to identify RNA (ribonucleic acid) sequences in the laboratory. First, fragments of RNA are separated using gel electrophoresis. Then, as in the Southern blot test, the fragments are covered with a nitrocellulose membrane. Lastly, a specific probe for this procedure is used to identify the RNA sequences present.

Important Terms

Accuracy: Accuracy refers to the ability of a test to obtain a true (or accurate) value.

Random Error: Random errors are any departures from the true or accurate value. Random errors are caused by errors that are inherent in all laboratory analyses and tests. The causes of random errors are often not able to be determined, and they are often unavoidable.

Precision: Precision is the reproducibility of results obtained from a particular test. If repeated testing provides the same results time after time, then there is said to be a high degree of precision.

Standard Deviation: The standard deviation is a value that estimates the random errors that are inherent in any test or analytical procedure. It gives insight into how much the obtained data values deviate from the mean (or average) data value.

Variance: The variance is the value of standard deviation multiplied by itself (square of the standard deviation). Similar to the standard deviation, it measures how obtained data values are spread around the mean (or average) value.

Mode: The mode is the particular numerical value that is the most frequent in a particular set of numbers.

Median: If a group of numbers are arranged from lowest to highest, according to magnitude, the median is the middle value of the set of numbers.

Geometric Mean: The geometric mean of a group of numbers is calculated by adding all of the logarithms of the numbers in the set of numbers divided by the quantity of numbers in the set. Then, the antilogarithm of this value is taken to obtain the geometric mean.

Arithmetic Mean: The arithmetic mean is usually called the average value. If you add up all of the numbers in a particular group of numbers, and then divide that result by the quantity of numbers in the group, the arithmetic mean is calculated.

Standard: A material, such as a serum, that has a known composition, and a high degree of purity. Standards are used to identify and describe other materials or samples. A standard is often described by its chemical and physical character. Laboratory standards are often available from the National Bureau of Standards.

Control: A control is a substance that contains known concentrations and amounts of the materials that will be measured in a particular test. The control will often have a chemical and physical character that is similar to sample being tested.

Coagulation: Formation of a clot. Four stage process: (1) damaged vessel constricts; (2) platelets adhere to damaged area (platelet adhesion) to form a platelet plug; (3) Extrinsic and intrinsic pathways lead to common pathway in which prothrombin activator reacts with calcium ions to form prothrombin, which forms thrombin, which causes fibrinogen to form fibrin monomers that react with fibrin stabilizing factor and calcium ions to form fibrin polymers that attract platelets and phospholipids to form a clot; (4) Fibrinolysis (clot breakdown) occurs when plasmin breaks fibrin into fragments, which are then removed by phagocytes.

Sodium citrate: Anticoagulant (crystalline compound) that prevents clotting but preserves coagulation factors.

Thrombin: Clot activator that converts fibrinogen into fibrin.

Platelet function test: Tests the ability of platelets to form a clot and helps to diagnose bleeding disorders.

Warfarin (Coumadin®): Warfarin (Coumadin®) is an anticoagulant that interferes with the formation of vitamin K–associated clotting factors (II, VII, IX, X) and C and S anticoagulant proteins.

FIFO ("first in, first out): Inventory is placed so that the oldest items are used first, especially important for items that are dated or perishable. This is the opposite of LIFO (last in, first out), which is used primarily for perishable items with a very limited shelf life.

Trigger level: AKA the reorder level (level at which replenishments must be ordered).

PAR (periodic automatic replenishment): The safety stock level, the minimum level to which the inventory can fall and still meet supply needs.

Standing order: Replenishments are provided on a regularly scheduled basis, such as every 2 weeks. Standard orders include the frequency and the quantity although this can be adjusted if necessary.

Expiration: Date by which an item is no longer usable, such as the expiration date on vacutainers.

Spectro-photometry: Measures absorption of light and quantity of coloring matter in a solution to determine composition. May be used to measure activity of enzymes, concentration of protein, bilirubin, glucose, and hemoglobin in serum.

Densitometry: Measures density of liquids and optical density in materials that are light sensitive. Used for DEXA bone scans.

Refractometry: Measures refractive index, how light goes through a substance, to identify composition and purity. Used to identify liquids, components, or characteristics, such as urine specific gravity and serum proteins.

Turbidimetry: Determines the concentration of solutions by how much light is absorbed by particles, which is dependent on the size and number of particles. Used to determine total protein, amylase activity, and lipase activity.

Nephelometry: Measures scattered light in a solution. Used to determine concentration of liquids with antigen-antibody reactions for a variety of lab tests, including immunoglobulins, serum proteins, hemoglobin, albumin, and C-reactive protein.

Osmometry: Measures osmolality of solution, compound, or colloid, such as serum or urine.

Chromatography: Uses a solid, gas, or liquid to separate a mixture into components in a 2-phase system (stationary and mobile) in which different components go through the medium at different speeds. Gas chromatography is used to detect drugs and alcohol in blood.

Mass spectrometry: Measures the masses found in a sample by converting molecules to ions and separating them and measuring and displaying them graphically. Used to analyze respiratory gases, genomic studies, and newborn screening.

Electrophoresis: Application of electric field to liquid applied to a medium to separate different macromolecules, such as proteins, RNA and DNA, by size and/or charge. Used for analysis of DNA, to determine the presence of proteins and antibody reactions, and to test antibiotics and vaccines.

Chemiluminescence: Light produced by a chemical reaction, such as when applying luminol to blood and observing under darkness. With a chemiluminescence assay, a light-emitting molecule is used to label an antigen or antibody in order to measure the antigen-antibody complex.

Enzyme-linked immunosorbent assay (ELISA): Plate-based assay utilizes antibodies and color to identify agents (such as antigens or antibodies). Used to determine the presence of antibodies to infections (such as HIV), allergens, hormones (pregnancy testing), or drugs (such as cocaine).

Fluorescence polarization immunoassay (FPIA): Antibody labeled with fluorescence and combined with a sample believed to contain an antigen and polarized light applied to identify and measure the amount of antigen that binds to the labeled antibody. Used for drug testing and therapeutic drug monitoring.

Prerenal: Classification of kidney disorders caused by problems outside of (before) the kidney, such as inadequate blood flow.

Suprapubic: Above the pubic bone, often the place where suprapubic catheters are placed, especially in males requiring long-term catheterization.

Glycosuria: Presence of glucose in the urine.

Renal threshold: The concentration at which the kidneys begin to remove a substance from the blood and into the urine.

Ascites: Accumulation of serous fluid in the abdominal cavity.

Tamm-Horsfall protein: AKA uromodulin, the most common protein found in normal urine.

Myoglobin: Protein found in muscle tissue.

Amniocentesis: Transabdominal sampling of amniotic fluid from the amniotic sac for prenatal diagnoses of chromosomal disorders and infections.

Pass-through: Duration of time that a drug needs to pass-through the liver and/or kidney.

Osmolality: Concentration of a substance (blood/urine).

Xanthochromic: Yellow-colored, usually in reference to cerebrospinal fluid that has the appearance of urine.

Carbohydrate: Class of nutrients comprised of carbon, hydrogen, and oxygen, and include simple carbohydrates (1 or 2 sugar molecules) or complex carbohydrates (multiple sugar molecules). Monosaccharides (1 sugar molecule) include glucose, fructose, and galactose. Disaccharides (2 linked monosaccharides) include sucrose, maltose, and lactose. Polysaccharides (thousands of linked glucose molecules) include starch, glycogen, and fiber, and do not taste sweet.

Ketones: Organic compound produced by the liver from fatty acids.

Lipogenesis: Metabolic process by which simple sugars are converted to fatty acids or triglycerides for storage.

Renal threshold (glucose): The glucose level at which the proximal tubule can no longer reabsorb glucose and it spills into the urine for excretion, usually when glucose levels reach 160-180 mg/dL.

Nucleated RBC (NRBC): Immature red blood cell that contain a nucleus, abnormal when found in peripheral blood.

Hematocrit: Percentage of erythrocytes in whole blood.

Reticulocyte: Immature erythrocyte that shows a basophilic reticulum under vital staining.

Hematopoiesis: Formation and maturation of blood cells.

Differential: Different types of leukocytes by percentage (monocytes, lymphocytes, neutrophils, basophils, and eosinophils).

Plasma: Liquid portion of blood or lymph.

Leukemia: Malignancy of blood-forming organs with abnormal proliferation and development of leukocytes and precursors.

Buffy coat: In centrifuged blood, the layer of leukocytes above the packed red blood cells.

Hypertonic: A solution with greater osmotic pressure than the solution to which it is compared.

Hypotonic: A solution with lower osmotic pressure than the solution to which it is compared.

Sodium citrate: Crystalline compound used as an anticoagulant and retains coagulation factors

Bacteria: Single-cell prokaryotic microorganisms that come in a variety of shapes, including coccus (spheres), bacillus (rods), spirals (DNA-like), and filamentous (elongated).

Capsule: The outside polysaccharide layer that surrounds some types of bacteria and protects the cell and provides a virulence factor.

Cytoplasm: Gel-like substance in the interior of the cell that comprises water, enzymes, various nutrients, waste products, and cell structures.

Nucleoid: Strands of DNA found in the cytoplasm.

Cell wall /Membrane: The cell wall is a subcapsular layer composed of peptidoglycan and is rigid to protect the underlying cytoplasmic membrane, which is composed of proteins and phospholipids that regulate the flow of substances to and from the cell. Composition varies among different bacteria. Gram-negative organisms have a thicker outer covering and gram-positive organisms have a thinner outer layer.

Spore: Resistant resting and/or reproductive stage of bacteria.

Flagella: Tail-like structure that helps control movement.

Pili: Hair-like projections that help bacteria attach to different surfaces, such as cells.

Facultative aerobic: Organism that prefers an environment without oxygen but has adapted to survive in the presence of oxygen. Examples include **Staphylococcus** spp. and **Lactobacillus.**

Microaerophilic aerobe: Organism that needs lower levels of oxygen than that typically found in the environment to survive and may also require higher levels of carbon dioxide. Examples include **Campylobacter** spp. and **Helicobacter pylori.**

Aerobic: Organism that lives and reproduces in an environment with oxygen. Obligate aerobes can only live in oxygenated environments. Example includes **Pseudomonas aeruginosa.**

Facultative anaerobic: Organism that is able to live and reproduce in an environment with or without oxygen. Examples include **Escherichia coli** and **Streptococcus** spp.

Anaerobic: Organism that lives and reproduces in an environment without oxygen. Obligate anaerobes can only live in the absence of oxygen. Example includes **Clostridium botulinum.**

Plasmapheresis: Form of hemapheresis in which plasma alone is removed from the blood of the donor; remaining blood products are returned to the donor, who may undergo this process once every eight weeks

Plateletpheresis: Only platelets are removed from donor blood; performed with an electronic apheresis instrument; donors may undergo this process once every 48 hours

Leukapheresis: White blood cells alone are removed from donor blood; performed with electronic apheresis instrument; donors may undergo this process no more than twice a week or 24 times in one year

Waived and Point-of-Care Testing

Waived Testing

While laboratory testing is regulated by CLIA and results monitored through proficiency testing, some tests are considered to have a very low risk of error (although not necessarily error free), and the patient is unlikely to experience harm if a result is in error. These tests do not require proficiency testing. **Waived testing** includes specific tests exempted by CLIA regulations, tests approved by the FDA for home use (such as pregnancy tests), and tests for which the FDA has applied a waiver based on CLIA regulations and guidelines. Labs that carry out only waived testing must obtain a CLIA Certificate of Waiver (COW). Waived tests include dipstick or tablet reagent tests (such as for bilirubin and ketones), fecal-occult blood tests, blood glucose monitoring strips, ovulation tests (color-based), ESR tests, blood counts, and hemoglobin. Some states may require proficiency testing for tests that are waived under CLIA regulations, and some laboratories may choose to have proficiency testing of waived tests for internal quality control.

Tests for Urinary Tract Infections

Urinary tract infections (UTIs) are infections that occur in some area of the urinary tract: kidneys, ureters, bladder, and/or urethra. Bladder infections (cystitis) are most common and are more frequent in females than males. Tests for urinary tract infections include:

- Microscopy: Urine sample is examined microscopically for evidence of infection, such as white blood cell, red blood cells, and casts.
- Urine culture: Used to determine the pathogenic agent causing the infection.
- Rapid urine test (point-of-care test): Enzymes produced by bacteria change nitrate into nitrite, which is measured as an indirect method to detect UTI. Urine must have been in bladder for at least 4 hours, so first morning sample is usually used. The rapid urine test also tests for a number of different substances: protein, glucose, ketones, bilirubin, urobilinogen, RBCs, WBCs as well as pH value. Procedure: Dip reagent strip in the urine sample and read results at 30 to 60 seconds and match against color chart with positive findings indicated by change to light to dark pink.

Common Coagulation Tests

Prothrombin time (PT)	10 – 14 seconds	Collect 1 mL blood in sodium citrate blue-capped tube (completely filled). Increased: Anticoagulation therapy, vitamin K deficiency, decreased prothrombin, DIC, liver disease, and malignant neoplasm. Some drugs may shorten time. Critical value: >27 seconds.
Partial thromboplastin time (PTT)	60-70 seconds	Collect 1 mL blood in sodium citrate blue-capped tube (completely filled). Increased: hemophilia A & B, von Willebrand's, vitamin deficiency, lupus, DIC, and liver disease. Critical value: >100 seconds.
Activated partial thromboplastin time (aPTT)	30-40 seconds	Collect 1 mL blood in sodium citrate blue-capped tube (completely filled). Similar to PTT but an activator added that speeds clotting time. Used to monitor heparin dosage. Increased: as for PTT. Decreased: Extensive cancer, early DIC, and after acute hemorrhage. Critical value: > 70 seconds.

D-Dimer	0.5 mcg/mL (measuring FEU*)	Collect 1 mL blood in sodium citrate blue-capped tube (completely filled) for immunoturbidimetry. Transport frozen. D-dimer is a specific polymer that results when fibrin breaks down, giving a marker to indicate the degree of fibrinolysis. Increased: DIC, pulmonary embolism, DVT, late pregnancy, neoplastic disorder, preeclampsia, arterial/venous thrombosis.

FEU = fibrinogen equivalent units

Point-of-Care Tests

Coagulation and Pregnancy

Point of care tests include:

- Coagulation: Point-of-care tests for coagulation use a sample of whole blood to provide the patient's PT, aPTT, and INR for patients on warfarin anticoagulant. Some devices can measure activated clotting time (ACT) for patients on unfractionated heparin. For example, the CoaguChek X is a handheld meter used to monitor INR. A sample of capillary blood is obtained and a drop of blood placed on a test strip. The test strip must be inserted into the device within 15 seconds. Coagulation measurement begins and the results are displayed. Test results for these devices are comparable to standard testing.
    - **INR:** (PT result/normal average): <2 for those not receiving anticoagulation and 2.0 to 3.0 those receiving anticoagulation. Critical value: >3-5 in patients receiving anticoagulation therapy.
- Pregnancy (human chorionic gonadotropin detection): Pregnancy tests are most accurate after a missed period and with the first morning urination. The patient should hold the testing stick in the stream of urine, or dip it in a cup of fresh urine. After the allotted wait time, the testing stick indicates whether the person is pregnant or not. False negatives may occur in early pregnancy.

Glucose

Point of care tests may give qualitative results (present or absent, such as pregnancy test) or quantitative result (precise numbers, such as glucose). Quality control is critical in ensuring that test results are accurate and those performing the tests must be well-trained. Advantages include rapid turnaround time and small sample volumes. Additionally, a sample does not require pre-processing. Disadvantages include increased cost, quality variation, and billing concerns. Tests include:

- Glucose: A glucometer is used with a drop of blood from a finger obtained with a lancet and applied to a strip and inserted into the properly calibrated glucometer, which reports the results. Normal values for a child range from 60 to 100 mg/dL and for an adult under 100 mg/dL (fasting usually ranges from 70 to 100). Critical values are less than 40 g/dL or greater than 400 mg/dL. Non-glucose sugars, such as those in peritoneal dialysate can affect results.

Hemoglobin and Hematocrit Testing

Hemoglobin	Hematocrit
Varies by age/gender.	Varies by age/gender.
Adult male: 13.2-17.3 g/dL	Adult male: 38 to 51%.
Adult female: 11.7-15.5 g/dL.	Adult female: 33 to 45%.
Critical values: <6.6 or >20 g/dL	Critical values (Adults): <19.8% or >60%.
Hemoglobin measures the amount of oxygen-carrying hemoglobin protein in the blood, and hematocrit measures the percentage of RBCs in whole blood.	

Hemoglobin	Hematocrit
Collection and purpose are the same: Whole blood is collected in lavender topped EDTA tube, Microtainer, or capillary tube or from green-topped lithium or sodium-heparin tube. The sample should be inverted 6-8 times immediately after blood draw. Test is done to assess anemia, hydration, polycythemia, and blood loss and to monitor therapy.	

Steps Taken When Quality Control Results Do Not Meet Acceptability Criteria

When new kits and reagents are used in the laboratory, control specimens must be tested to ensure quality. If **quality control results** do not meet acceptability criteria, then no further testing or reporting of results can be done until the problem is resolved and accurate testing is ensured. Quality control specimens may be internal (part of the kit), external (outside of the kit), or electronic. If results are not accurate, the following steps should be carried out:

- Review the package insert to ensure all directions were carried out correctly and read through any "troubleshooting" information.
- Verify expiration dates on all materials utilized for testing.
- Verify that all solutions and supplies were properly stored, including at the appropriate temperature and light exposure.
- Verify that the specimen type is correct.
- Review procedures to ensure that mixing and preparation was carried out correctly.
- Check to make sure that all equipment has been properly cleaned and prepared.
- Run the test with another quality control specimen.
- Carefully document all steps taken to correct the problem.

Laboratory Operations

Various Agencies and Their Responsibilities

National Accrediting Agency for Clinical Laboratory Sciences - The agency responsible for approving and accrediting clinical laboratory science and similar healthcare professional education programs.

College of American Pathologists - The primary organization for board-certified pathologists serving to represent the interests of the public, as well as pathologists and their patients by fostering excellence in the pathology and laboratory medicine practice.

The Joint Commission - A large organization that aims to improve the quality of care provided to patients through implementing healthcare accreditation standards and other supportive services aimed at improving the performance of healthcare organizations.

AHA's Patient Care Partnership

The American Hospital Association developed the **Patient Care Partnership** as a replacement for the Patient's Bill of Rights. It outlines what patients have a right to expect during hospitalization in relation to their rights and responsibilities:

- High quality hospital care: Patient should know identity of caregivers and their positions (physician, nurse, student, therapist) and should be able to express concerns about care.
- Clean, safe environment: Care should be free of abuse or neglect and provided in a clean, safe environment.
- Involvement in care: Patient should participate in the plan of care, give informed consent, and be provided information about whether treatments are experimental or part of research and should understand long-term effects of treatment, discharge expectations, and financial consequences of services. The patient needs to provide complete and accurate information about history, medicines, health plan, and advance directives.
- Protection of privacy: Patient should receive a Notice of Privacy.
- Help with bills and filing insurance claims: Staff will file claims and provide information to patient.
- Discharge planning for patient and family: Patient advised of resources and follow-up medications and treatments.

OSHA and SDS

OSHA stands for Occupational Safety and Health Administration. It is an organization designed to assure the safety and health of workers by setting and enforcing standards; providing training, outreach, and education; establishing partnerships; and encouraging continual improvement in workplace safety and health. SDS (formerly MSDS) stands for Safety Data Sheets. These sheets are the result of the "Right to Know" Law also known as the OSHA's HazCom Standard. This law requires chemical manufacturers to supply SDS sheets on any products that have a hazardous warning label. These sheets contain information on precautionary as well as emergency information about the product.

Review Video: Intro to OSHA
Visit mometrix.com/academy and enter code: 913559

OSHA Regulations Regarding Laboratory Services

The **Occupational Safety and Health Administration** (OSHA) requires that facilities provide safe medical equipment and devices. OSHA also regulates workplace safety, including disposal methods for sharps, such as needles, and blood disposition. OSHA requires that standard precautions be used at all times and that staff be trained to use precautions. OSHA requires procedures for post-exposure evaluation and treatment and availability of hepatitis B vaccine for healthcare workers. OSHA defines occupational exposure to infections, establishes standards to prevent the spread of bloodborne pathogens, and regulates the fitting and use of respirators. OSHA (Occupational Safety and Health Administration) requires the use of needleless blood transfer devices as a means of decreasing the risk of needlestick injuries and infection as part of OSHA's Bloodborne Pathogen Standard. Sharps used for blood draw should have sharps injury protection devices whenever possible. Needles without this protection should never be recapped as this increases risk of needlestick. States may have their own OSHA-approved programs but must meet the minimum standards developed by OSHA.

Risk Management

Risk Management is a system that involves identifying and reducing situations that pose unnecessary risk to employees or patients by following specific procedures and by adequately educating employees on policies and procedures adopted by the facility.

Quality Control

Quality Control is a series of checks and control measures that ensure that a uniform excellence of service is provided

Quality Assurance

The system utilizing quality reviews of services and the taking of any corrective actions to remove or improve any deficiencies

Polypropylene

Polypropylene is a type of plastic. Polypropylene is rigid, translucent, and it has a non-wettable surface, similar to Teflon. Polypropylene can also be autoclaved, because it has a melting point of 320 degrees Fahrenheit (160 degrees Celsius). This high melting point makes polypropylene able to withstand the high temperatures of an autoclave. In the laboratory, most pipette tips are made out of polypropylene, as are some test tubes and diluent trays.

Polycarbonate

Polycarbonate is another type of plastic. Sometimes, polycarbonate goes by the trademark name, Nalgene. Polycarbonate plastics are flexible, lightweight, and strong. They are able to withstand high impacts without breaking upon impact. In the laboratory, they can be used as a substitute for glass, because of their shatter-resistant capabilities.

Polyvinylchloride (PVC)

Polyvinylchloride, or PVC, is a type of plastic. Polyvinylchloride is clear, can either be flexible or rigid, and it can also be either non-autoclavable or autoclavable. Flexible, autoclavable polyvinylchloride is used to make plastic tubing for use in the laboratory. This tubing can be used in various pieces of automated laboratory equipment, including continuous flow analyzers. Polyvinylchloride that is rigid and non-autoclavable is used to make plastic bottles for laboratory use.

Polytetrafluoroethylene

Polytetrafluoroethylene is a compound that sometimes goes by its trademark, Teflon. Teflon is a compound that has a slippery surface, and it is tough and stable over a wide range of temperatures It also has a non-wettable surface. In the laboratory, Teflon is used to make transfer disks for centrifugal analyzers, and it is also used to make stoppers and gaskets.

Kimax and Corex Glass

Kimax is a brand name for borosilicate glass. Borosilicate glasses contain at least 5% boric acid in their composition. They are also made up of sodium oxide, potassium oxide, calcium oxide, and silica. Borosilicate glasses are very heat resistant and strong as well. They also have a low thermal expansion coefficient, meaning that they do not expand much when heated. In the laboratory, flasks, beakers, and pipettes are usually made of borosilicate glass. Pyrex is another brand name of borosilicate glass products.

Corex is a brand name for aluminum-silicate glass. Aluminum-silicate glass is even stronger than borosilicate glass -- about six times stronger. Aluminum silicate glass also exhibits resistance to scratching and etching from alkaline materials. Corex glass is used in the laboratory in the form of thermometers and centrifuge tubes.

Desiccant

A desiccant is a material that readily absorbs water (hygroscopic). Desiccants are used to keep things dry and to prevent them from becoming hydrated or in contact with water. In the laboratory, some things that desiccants are used to keep dry are reagents, gases used in gas chromatography, and thin-layer chromatography (TLC) plates. Usually, a desiccator is used. A desiccator is typically made out of glass, and the material in question is placed on a small shelf, with the desiccant placed below the shelf. A glass lid makes an air tight seal on the vessel. Some of the materials that can be used as desiccants include silica gel, calcium sulfate, sodium hydroxide, and magnesium perchloride. One of the least effective desiccants is silica gel, and the most effective desiccant is magnesium perchloride.

Regulatory Bodies Governing Coding and Billing

CPT codes, developed by the American Medical Association (AMA), define those licensed to provide services and describe medical and surgical treatments, diagnostics, and procedures done on an outpatient basis. The use of CPT codes is mandated by both CMS and HIPAA to provide a uniform language and to aid research. These codes are used primarily for billing purposes for insurances (public and private). HHS has designed CPT codes as part of the national standard for electronic healthcare transactions:

- Category I: Identify a procedure or service.
- Category II: Identify performance measures, including diagnostic procedures.
- Category III: Identify temporary codes for technology and data collection.

ICD-10 codes are the tenth version of the WHO's International Statistical Classification of Diseases and Related Health Problems (ICD) codes and include ICD-10-CM, which codes for diagnosis, and ICD-10-PCS, which codes for inpatient procedures. ICD codes were developed by the World Health Organization. Use of these codes is mandated by CMS. Because insurance companies use the same coding systems as CMS, these codes are used across healthcare.

Universal Precautions

Universal precautions are used in the laboratory and other medical settings to help protect healthcare workers from diseases and poisons transmitted via bodily fluids and secretions (blood, semen, amniotic fluid, vaginal secretions, sweat, tears, saliva, urine, feces, wound drainage and CSF). Universal precautions became required practice after the outbreak of AIDS in 1980. Universal precautions means washing thoroughly and wearing protective gear, such as gloves, goggles or glasses, face shields, shoe covers, gowns, and anything else deemed appropriate by Infection Control. Which precautions need to be practiced in a given situation depend on the possibility of a healthcare worker coming in contact with the bodily fluids or secretions, not on the patient's known health status. Assume all patients are always infectious.

WHO Rules for Laboratory Safety

Each laboratory must have a manual that contains safety regulations. Labs should have sufficient workspace and accommodate disabled workers. Areas with patient access should be separate from the work area. The World Health Organization (WHO) has established rules for **laboratory safety**:

- The laboratory must be separate from areas of unrestricted traffic flow.
- Entry to the laboratory should be through double doors or a vestibule.
- All surfaces should be water-resistant for easy cleaning and well sealed, impervious to water, and resistant to chemicals, such as acids and solvents.
- The laboratory itself must be sealable and allow for gaseous decontamination.
- Windows must be kept closed and sealed, and must be resistant to breakage.
- Airflow must be into the laboratory from access rooms.
- Negative pressure airflow must be maintained and intake and output filtered through a HEPA filter. Output must be discharged outside of the building and at a distance from air intakes.
- The water supply must be outfitted with anti-backflow devices.
- All effluent must be decontaminated before discharged into the sewer system.
- Biological safety cabinets must have a negative airflow filter.

Equipment Safety

Equipment safety is essential because lancets, needles, and other sharp objects pose risks to laboratory personnel and must be used properly and disposed of safely in specific ("sharps") containers designed for safety. Procedures should be in place for all use of sharps and standard precautions followed. Safety lancets with needles that automatically retract should be utilized if possible. Safety needles are also available; if using a standard needle, the needle should not be recapped or bent prior to disposal but placed directly into the container, sharp end downward. Sharps containers should be leak-proof, resistant to punctures, clearly labeled, and placed in a convenient place not accessible by children. Most sharps containers are red, but clear containers may also be used so it is easier to see when they are full. Containers should never be filled to the top because of the risk that a needle or other sharp item may protrude through the opening.

Proper Storage of Chemicals

Proper storage of chemicals in the laboratory is vital to maintaining technician safety and a safe work place. All lab chemicals must have the proper labels and be stored in the proper container. For example, materials that are flammable need to be stored in a fire safety cabinet, to minimize the risk of fire. Solvents, on the other hand, need to be stored in a refrigerator that is explosion-proof. In addition to using proper storage containers and equipment, chemicals that are incompatible with each other should never be stored together. An example of this would be storing oxidizing agents next to reducing agents. Therefore, chemicals should never be stored alphabetically, as this may place incompatible chemicals next to each other in a storage situation. The amount of flammable substances and solvents that are stored should be limited, further reducing the risk of fire. Store large containers on a low shelf, close to the ground, to minimize dangers if these containers break. Check storage areas monthly to make sure that everything is stored properly.

Safety Precautions When Collecting Blood Samples

Safety precautions when collecting blood samples include:

- Plan ahead and ensure all needed supplies are on hand.
- Wear a lab coat that is fully buttoned to protect clothing.
- Carry out proper hand hygiene before and after procedures.
- Wear gloves for phlebotomy procedures and any processing.
- Follow standard precautions throughout the procedure.

- Utilize safety-engineered devices, such as retractable needles and lancets, and single-use devices when possible.
- Do not recap or bend needles prior to disposal.
- If recapping of a needle is necessary, use one-hand scooping method.
- Dispose of needles and syringes as one unit rather than separating.
- Dispose of sharps in appropriate containers.
- Ensure immunization for hepatitis B is current.
- Immediately report any exposure to blood or body fluids and begin PEP if needed.
- Ensure the work area for collection is well lighted and clean.
- Follow protocols for blood collection.
- Obtain assistance for unruly or confused patients.
- Place sample tube in rack prior to injecting sample through rubber stopper.

Proper Infection Control

Each laboratory should carry out a biological risk assessment each year or when new risks arise to determine the biosafety level and agent hazards and procedures hazards. Work practices should conform to Bloodborne Pathogen Standard (Occupational Safety and Health Administration [OSHA]) and standard precautions (CDC). **Infection control** precautions include:

- Utilizing appropriate hand hygiene with hand-free sink for washing hands available near exit.
- Using mechanical pipettes instead of mouth pipetting.
- Eating, drinking, smoking, storing food, applying makeup, and handling contact lenses all prohibited in the laboratory.
- Maintaining safe handling of sharps policies.
- Utilizing safety devices (retractable needles, lances) when possible.
- Minimizing splashing or aerosolizing liquids.
- Decontaminating potentially infectious materials prior to disposal.
- Packing potentially infectious materials for disposal outside of facility in appropriate packaging according to regulations.
- Maintaining a pest management program.
- Ensuring that all personnel are adequately trained.
- Ensuring appropriate immunizations and screening for personnel.
- Making PPE available and monitoring appropriate use.
- Ensuring eye wash station is easily accessed and available.

Laws Governing Reportable Incidents

The Occupational Safety and Health Administration (OSHA) has established regulations and guidelines for laboratory safety through the OSHA Laboratory Standard. According to these guidelines, laboratory employees must report all incidents, equipment malfunctions, and work-related injuries and illnesses to a supervisor. Work-related exposures/injuries/illnesses (CFR 29-1904) that must be reported include:

1. Muscle strains and contusions.
2. Lacerations or puncture injuries.
3. Needlestick injuries.
4. Chemical exposure: spills, splashing.
5. Infectious agent exposure.
6. Burns.
7. Death.

An incident report must be filled out for all work-related exposure/injuries and those needing medical attention are covered by Workers' Compensation. Work-related injuries must be reported on the OSHA

300 Log if the case meets general recording criteria, which includes death, one or more calendar days in which the person was unable to work (beginning with the day after the injury and counting days that the person was not scheduled to work up to 180 days), loss of consciousness, medical treatment beyond first aid, significant injury or illness (diagnosed by licensed healthcare provider), and the need for restricted work or transfer because of the injury.

Quality Control Procedures Based on CLSI Standards

The **Clinical and Laboratory Standards Institute** (CLSI) provides standards for a wide range of performance and testing and cover all types of laboratory functions and microbiology. These standards are used as a basis for quality control procedures. Standards include:

1. Labeling: The label must be 2 inches × 1 inch and contain the required elements (patient name (left upper corner), unique identifier, birth date, date and time of collection, and collector's signature or ID.
2. Security/Information technology: Technical operational and implementation requirements for *in vitro* analytical equipment and data management must be followed and essential elements included and de-identification practices utilized.
3. Toxicology/Drug testing: Protocols for collecting, analyzing, interpreting, and reporting results of drug testing should be used as the basis for development of procedures.
4. Statistical quality control/Quantitative measurements: Provides guidance for quality control of different measurement procedures to ensure accuracy and safety of laboratory personnel.
5. Performance standards for various types of antimicrobial susceptibility testing.

Quality Control

As part of **quality control**, only personnel who are properly trained and qualified through education should be employed in the laboratory. Measures to ensure quality control include:

- Checking speed of centrifuge, volumes dispensed by diluters, temperature of water baths, and proper storage and expiration dates of reagents.
- Checking for proper instrument handling.
- Ensuring that appropriate organisms are used for sensitivity testing.
- Double-checking negative reports (especially in parasitology) by supervising personnel.
- Evaluating processing time to ensure samples are tested within the appropriate window, such as 2 hours for urine specimens and 4 hours for white blood cell counts.
- Correlating results, such as reviewing both hemoglobin and hematocrit.
- Maintaining accurate and appropriate records.
- Preparing a quality control chart.
- Establishing standards and controls for daily laboratory operation.
- Establishing standards and protocols for acceptance or rejection of samples and analysis.
- Applying Westgard's rule to determine acceptable variation in control before rejecting test results.
- Determining if a run has occurred to indicate results are out of control and should be rejected.

Laws and Laboratory Regulations

In the United States, all laboratory testing, except for research, is regulated by the CMS (Centers for Medicare and Medicaid Services) through **Clinical Laboratory Improvement Amendments (CLIA).** CLIA is implemented through the Division of Laboratory Services and serves approximately 244,000 laboratories. Laboratories receiving reimbursement from CMS must meet CLIA standards, which ensure that laboratory testing will be accurate and procedures followed properly. The Centers for Disease Control and Prevention (CDC) partners with CMS and the Food and Drug Administration (FDA) in supporting CLIA programs. Physician office laboratories are most often accredited by COLA (Commission on Laboratory Accreditation), founded in 1988 with the original intent of inspecting and accrediting physician office laboratories to ensure that they were in compliance with CLIA. COLA has since expanded its mission and now also accredits hospital laboratories as well as independent laboratories. CMS and the Joint Commission have granted deeming authority to COLA.

Proficiency Testing

Proficiency testing is a method of quality control that assesses the performance (accuracy and reliability) of a laboratory in carrying out tests and measurements, comparing laboratory results with those of other laboratories. Samples that have been previously tested by reference laboratories to establish reference values are sent to the laboratory by a CMS-approved proficiency testing agency for blind testing and the results are checked against those obtained by the reference laboratories. Samples are generally sent to participating laboratories about every 4 months with 5 samples sent each time with at least 1 sample specific to the type of testing the lab carries out, such as gram stains and organism identification. Testing must be carried out on the samples in the same manner as actual patient specimens, and samples may not be forwarded to other laboratories for testing or to verify results. The results are submitted to the proficiency testing agency, which grades the findings and sends the laboratory a score. Both CMS and accreditation agencies routinely monitor these scores.

Quality Improvement

TQM

Total Quality Management (TQM) is one philosophy of quality management that espouses a commitment to meeting the needs of the customers at all levels within an organization. It promotes not only continuous improvement but also a dedication to quality in all aspects of an organization. Outcomes should include increased customer satisfaction and productivity, as well as increased profits through efficiency and reduction in costs. In order to provide TQM, an organization must seek the following:

- Information regarding customer's needs and opinions.
- Involvement of staff at all levels in decision making, goal setting, and problems solving.
- Commitment of management to empowering staff and being accountable through active leadership and participation.
- Institution of teamwork with incentives and rewards for accomplishments.

The focus of TQM is on working together to identify and solve problems rather than assigning blame through an organizational culture that focuses on the needs of the customers.

CQI

Continuous Quality Improvement (CQI) emphasizes the organization and systems and processes within that organization rather than individuals. It recognizes internal customers (staff) and external customers (patients) and utilizes data to improve processes. CQI represents the concept that most processes can be improved. CQI uses the scientific method of experimentation to meet needs and improve services and utilizes various tools, such as brainstorming, multivoting, various charts and diagrams, storyboarding, and meetings. Core concepts include:

- Quality and success is meeting or exceeding internal and external customer's needs and expectations.
- Problems relate to processes, and variations in process lead to variations in results.
- Change can be in small steps.

Steps to CQI include:

- Forming a knowledgeable team.
- Identifying and defining measures used to determine success.
- Brainstorming strategies for change.

- Plan, collect, and utilize data as part of making decisions.
- Test changes and revise or refine as needed.

PIC

The **Performance Improvement Council (PIC)** was developed by the US government (Title 31, Code 1124) as an interagency collaborative effort to share information in order to improve performance and management, although the principles of openness and sharing can also be applied to the private sector. Members of the PIC include performance improvement officers as well as representatives from various federal agencies and departments. These members of the central PIC work together to facilitate communication and share best practices by providing consultation services and facilitators to help others develop cross-agency teams and establish priority goals. The PIC actively seeks information regarding best practices from both governmental and private sector entities. Each governmental agency must assign a performance improvement officer whose responsibility is to improve performance and coordinate with interagency councils. The PIC is active in setting goals as well as measurement and analysis, including performance review and capacity building.

Preanalytical, Analytical, and/or Postanalytical Causes of Erroneous Results

Erroneous results may occur because of problems in any step in the collection and processing of specimens, but the greatest danger of errors occurs in the preanalytical stage, where many different things can go wrong:

- Preanalytical errors: Include hemolysis of specimen, inappropriate request for test, error in order entry, inadequate sample volume/size, use of incorrect tube, improper identification of patient, improper preservation method for specimen, tube breakage (before or during centrifugation), inadequate centrifugation (time/speed), delayed transport, reagent expired, ID or barcode unclear, duplicate pathological numbers, and specimens mixed up.
- Analytical errors: Include quality control failure and malfunctioning of equipment resulting in improper results.
- Postanalytical errors: Include failure to post results, error in interpretation of results, excessive turnaround time, and failure to collect results.

Quality Assurance Measures Related to Autoclaving

Quality assurance testing of an autoclave determines if an autoclave can reach a correct temperature for a long enough period of time, usually 121 degree Celsius for fifteen minutes. Striped tape and chemical indicators are used. A color change will indicate when the temperature and time conditions have been reached. Physical indicators, such as a melting metal alloy, can also indicate that the required conditions have been met. A biological indicator, a suspension containing spores of *Bacillus stearothermophilus*, can also be used. This particular bacterium is heat resistant, so if the required autoclave conditions have not been met, the spores will germinate, and deteriorate the glucose that is present in the suspension. Color changes from purple to yellow. However, if the autoclave conditions have been met, spores will not germinate, and there will be no viable spores visible after an incubation period of seven days at 55 degrees Celsius, and no color change.

Manual Instrumentation

Borosilicate glassware is heat and chemical resistant; soda lime glassware, less expensive and less resistant; and plastic ware, less expensive and less breakable but not heat resistant and cannot be used with some reagents and chemicals. Commonly used **manual laboratory instrumentation** includes:

- Test tubes: Used to heat and hold reagents to assess chemical reactions. Vary in size and usually rimless. Held in plastic or metal test tube racks. Centrifuge tubes (15 mL) are similar but have tapered ends to hold pellet. Cuvettes are rectangular test tubes to hold solutions for photometry, placed only in plastic racks to avoid scratching.

- Funnels (plain and separating): Supported in ring stand and used for filtration or to separate immiscible liquids.
- General purpose and volumetric glassware: Includes graduated cylinders, volumetric flasks, pipettes, and burettes and used for measuring volumes. Pipettes or eyedroppers are used to transfer liquids. Mouth pipettes should never be used. Reagent bottles hold reagents. Beakers are used to heat liquids.

Automated Laboratory Instrumentation

Automated laboratory instrumentation is becoming the norm, and a laboratory may have total laboratory automation or system-based automation. Automated laboratory instrumentation has a number of advantages over manual procedures:

- Test results can be obtained faster and are often more accurate because they are not dependent on varying techniques and subjective judgment.
- Test results are more reliable and consistent, and can be easily reproduced.
- Data can be more easily stored, transferred, manipulated, and reported.
- Fewer laboratory personnel are needed because the automated systems can do the work of many technicians.
- Errors are minimized.
- Workflow is more efficient.

However, there are also some disadvantages: If a machine breaks down, there may be considerable delay in manually producing lab reports because of inadequate staffing or equipment. Additionally, staff members must be trained in trouble shooting and maintenance of equipment and service technicians must be available. The automation equipment may be prohibitively expensive, especially for a small laboratory.

Calibration of Instruments

Generally, all instruments used to generate, measure, and assess data should be routinely calibrated and tested, based on standards and standard operating procedures. The frequency may vary, but some require daily **calibration** while others need calibration every few months. Equipment should also be calibrated if mechanical or other problems have occurred. Calibration may be done manually or semi- or completely automatically, and procedures may vary, but usually include:

- Testing calibrators, solutions, or samples with known values, to determine accuracy of measurement.
- Carefully preparing calibrators, including correct volumes.
- Following directions exactly (according to manufacturer's guidelines), maintaining the proper conditions (light, heat, ventilation), and using calibrators in the correct order and manner.
- Noting the need for adjustments to the equipment or process.

Calibration is part of quality control, but those instruments, supplies, or equipment that are not involved in directly generating, measuring, or assessing data generally do not require calibration but are maintained as part of general quality control.

Centrifuges

Centrifuges spin solutions to separate out solid materials by forcing them away from the center to form a pellet. Centrifuges come in various sizes and may be free floating/horizontal or angle-head (45-degree angle). Different specimens require different G-forces/relative centrifugal force (RCF) (which is the spinning force relative to earth's gravitation) and different durations. The G-force/RCF depends on the revolutions per minute (RPMs) and the radius of revolution (RR) (measured in mm from the center to the end of the test tube): RCF/G-force = 1.12 × RR × $(RPM/1000)^2$ (or use nomogram chart). Procedure:

- Use equal numbers of tubes in the buckets on opposite sites. Weigh tubes to ensure the load is balanced and use a tube filled with water if testing an odd number.
- Close and lock centrifuge, turn it on, and follow instructions for settings.
- Spin for necessary duration (such as 15 to 20 minutes). If excessive vibration (from imbalance) or sound of cracking vial occurs, turn off machine.
- When completed, remove buckets carefully to avoid jarring the pellets.
- Open buckets and remove tubes, checking for sediments.

Microscopes

The **microscope** most commonly used is the light microscope (either monocular or binocular). This microscope uses external light or light from an internal filament that allows the light to pass upward through the specimen so that the specimen appears dark against the lighter background, although the light may be inverted, illuminating from the top, for such things as a culture in a liquid medium. Phase contrast microscopes that do not require staining of the specimen are used to assess cell growth, especially for organisms that are transparent with standard light microscope. The dark field microscope uses a special dark-field condenser that makes the specimen appear light against a dark background, useful for observing spirochetes. The fluorescent microscope utilizes an ultraviolet light for illumination. This microscope is used when fluorescent dye is attached to a specimen because the dye glows when exposed to ultraviolet light, useful for fluorescent antibody testing.

Calibration of Ocular Micrometers

The ocular micrometer is a glass disk that fits into the microscope eyepiece and provides an engraved ruler for measurement within the ocular lens. The **ocular micrometer calibration** procedure is as follows:

- Remove eyepiece and unscrew the ocular eye lens and position the ocular micrometer with the engraved ruler with 100 divisions face down, replace the lens, and place the ocular with the micrometer into the ocular tube and microscope with 10× objective.
- Place a stage micrometer slide with an engraved scale that closely matches in the ocular micrometer length and number of divisions on the microscope stage and focus on the parallel sets of rulers so that the 0-mm lines on the ocular micrometer and stage micrometer align.
- Locate another set of lines that align at the furthest distance from the 0-mm lines.
- Count the number of lines between the 0-mm alignment and the distant alignment on both the ocular micrometer scale and the stage micrometer scale.
- Use formulas to determine the proportion of a mm measured by 1 ocular unit:
- Stage micrometer reading × 1000 micrometers/ocular micrometer reading × 1 mm = ocular units.
- For 40× objective: 0.1 mm × 1000 micrometer/50 units × 1 mm.

Computer Hardware and Software

Computer hardware consists of all of the physical parts of a computer. All machinery and equipment that makes up the computer and its related components are considered hardware. This includes computer disks, cables, the CPU (central processing unit), printers, keyboard, modem, and any other physical parts of the computer. A computer's hardware is what indicates what a computer is capable of doing.

Computer software, on the other hand, is all of the programs that tell a computer how to operate. Software can be divided into application software, which are programs that manipulate and process data, and system software, which control the computer and other programs. Software is written in various programming languages, and the software is responsible for controlling what the hardware does and how the hardware operates.

Benefits of Computerized Data Automation in Laboratories

Computerized automation of laboratory data has several advantages. For one, with the computer taking care of recording and storing data, laboratory technicians have more time to do other clinical tasks, such as performing laboratory tests. This increases laboratory productivity. Data stored on a computer, instead of paper laboratory reports, requires less storage space and can be encrypted for confidentiality. Another reason that computer automation is beneficial is that with data stored in a computer system, doctors and nurses can access such data much faster than if paper reports had to be mailed or faxed to them. In some cases, doctors can log onto a hospital computer system to see test results right away. And, using a computer to record data leads to fewer filing and billing errors on the part of the laboratory technicians.

Ordering Sets of Data Measurements from Lowest to Highest Memory

Example

Order the following sets of data measurements measurements in order of lowest to highest memory:

5 characters, 1 Kbyte, 20 bytes, 16,000 bits

24,000 bits, 1000 characters, 500 bytes, 4 Kbyte

The following conversions are helpful for this problem: 1 character = 1 byte; 1 byte = 8 bits; 1 Kbyte = 1024 bytes.

1. In this situation, it would be helpful to convert everything to one common unit, such as bytes. So, 5 characters = 5 bytes; 1 Kbyte = 1024 bytes; 16,000 bits = 2000 bytes. 20 bytes does not need to be converted. Therefore, in order from lowest to highest memory, the order is: 5 characters, 20 bytes, 1Kbyte, 16,000 bits.
2. In this situation, it would be helpful again to convert everything to one common unit, such as bytes. So, 24,000 bits = 3000 bytes; 1000 characters = 1000 bytes; 4 Kbyte = 4096 bytes. 500 bytes does not need to be converted. Therefore, in order from lowest to highest memory, the order is: 500 bytes, 1000 characters, 24,000 bits, 4 Kbyte.

Maintaining Security of Laboratory Computers and Databases

Security of laboratory computers and databases is a very important issue in the medical laboratory. Patient confidentiality must be kept at all times, and patients' data must not get into the wrong hands or be viewed by the wrong set of eyes. Because of this, there are various methods that laboratories can use to keep their computers and databases safe. Using passwords and identification numbers or names for each laboratory technician or doctor is a widely used method for security. Also, limiting the access to the computers can help as well. Using voice recognition technologies or keys that must be inserted into locks on the computers can keep computers and data safe. Various software programs, such as anti-virus, anti-spyware, and encryption software can enhance security. It must be noted, however, that security measures should not greatly impact the ease of using the computers.

Molarity of a Solution

The molarity (M) of a solution is equal to moles per liter.

EXAMPLE

Determine the molarity (M) of a solution that contains 20.0 grams of NaCl in 500 mL of solution.

The molarity (M) of a solution is equal to moles per liter. In this example, we need to calculate what one mole (gram molecular weight) is of NaCl first. A mole of a compound is equal to the sum of the atomic weights of the elements in that compound. So, for NaCl, one mole is equal to the atomic weight of Na plus the atomic weight of Cl (23.0g + 35.5g), or 58.5 g. Next, it is best to determine the concentration of the solution in terms of grams per liter. So, in our example, the solution is 20.0 g NaCl/500 mL. This is equivalent to 20.0g NaCl/0.5 L, or 40g NaCl/L. Next, the number of moles of NaCl present in the solution must be calculated. Take the grams of NaCl present in 1 liter of solution and divide it by the weight of one mole of NaCl (40g NaCl/58.5g NaCl). In our example, the number of moles present is therefore equal to 0.68 moles. Since molarity is equal to moles per liter, the molarity of this solution is therefore 0.68 mol/L, or the solution is a 0.68 M NaCl solution.

CONVERTING BETWEEN FAHRENHEIT AND CELSIUS

EXAMPLES

Perform the following conversions:

1. 55 degrees Fahrenheit to degrees Celsius
2. 32 degrees Fahrenheit to degrees Celsius
3. 12 degrees Celsius to degrees Fahrenheit
4. 31 degrees Celsius to degrees Fahrenheit

ANSWERS

1. To convert from degrees Fahrenheit to degrees Celsius, the following equation is used: degrees Celsius = (degrees Fahrenheit - 32) x 5/9. Plugging in the number given for degrees Fahrenheit, 55, the degrees Celsius is calculated to be approximately 13 degrees.
2. To convert from degrees Fahrenheit to degrees Celsius, the following equation is used: degrees Celsius = (degrees Fahrenheit – 32) x 5/9. Using the number given for degrees Fahrenheit, 32, the degrees Celsius is calculated to be 0 degrees.
3. To convert from degrees Celsius to degrees Fahrenheit, the following equation is used: degrees Fahrenheit = (degrees Celsius x 9/5) + 32. Plugging in the number given for degrees Celsius, 12, the degrees Fahrenheit is calculated to be approximately 54 degrees.
4. To convert from degrees Celsius to degrees Fahrenheit, the following equation is used: degrees Fahrenheit = (degrees Celsius x 9/5) + 32. Plugging in the number given for degrees Celsius, 31, the degrees Fahrenheit is calculated to be approximately 88 degrees.

BEER'S LAW

Beer's law is defined as $A = abc$, where A is the absorbance, *a* is the absorptivity, *b* is the path of light in centimeters (cm), and *c* is the concentration of the absorbing compound.

EXAMPLE

For a certain spectrophotometric procedure, the absorbance of a standard solution (concentration is 25 mg/dL) is 0.75 (in a 1 cm cell). The absorbance of the sample solution is 0.35 (in a 1 cm cell). Calculate the concentration of the sample solution.

For the problem given, both b (the path of light in centimeters) and a (the absorptivity) are constant. So, using Beer's law, the equation then becomes: $c_{sample}/c_{standard} = A_{sample}/A_{standard}$. All of the values in that equation are known except for the concentration of the sample, c_{sample}. Rearranging the equation gives: $c_{sample} = A_{sample}/A_{standard} \times c_{standard}$.

Plugging in the values given in the problem gives the following: c_{sample} = 0.35/0.75 x 25 mg/dL or 11.7 mg/dL. 11.7 mg/dL is the concentration of the sample solution.

Osmolality

Osmolality is defined as the moles per 1 kilogram (kg) of solvent multiplied by the number of particles into which the molecules of solute dissociate.

Example

Calculate the osmolality of 54 g glucose and 11.7 g NaCl in 2 kg of water.

To calculate the osmolality in the given problem, first we need to calculate how many moles of solute (both glucose and NaCl) are present. For glucose, 54 g of glucose = 54 g/180 g/mol = 0.3 mol glucose. For NaCl, 11.7 g NaCl = 11.7 g/58.5 g/mol = 0.2 mol NaCl. Then, we need to look at how each solute dissociates. Glucose does not really dissociate well. However, 0.2 mol of NaCl will dissociate into two particles, 0.2 mol of Na^+ and 0.2 mol of Cl^-. So, to calculate the number of Osmoles present, we would add 0.3 Osmole of glucose to 0.2 Osmole of Na^+ and 0.2 Osmole of Cl^-. This totals 0.7 Osmoles present. Because we are dealing with 2 kg of water, however, and osmolality is noted as moles per 1 kilogram, we need to divide 0.7 Osmoles by 2 kg of water, to give 0.35 Osmoles per 1 kg of water, or 0.35 Osmolal.

Calculating Concentration of Milliequivalents Per Liter

To calculate a concentration in milliequivalents per liter (mEq/L), when given concentration in milligrams per deciliter (mg/dL), the following equation needs to be used:

(mg/dL x 10 dL/L x valence) / atomic mass = mEq/L.

Examples

Calculate the concentration in milliequivalents per liter (mEq/L) of each of the following:

1. serum potassium level of 22.3 mg/dL
2. serum calcium level of 9.0 mg/dL

1. For potassium, the valence of potassium is 1, and the atomic mass of potassium is 39. These values can be obtained by using a periodic table. Therefore, the equation then becomes (22.3 mg/dL x 10 dL/L x 1) / 39 = 5.7 mEq/L.
2. For this example, we can use the same equation as in part a to calculate mEq/L; (mg/dL x 10 dL/L x valence) / atomic mass = mEq/L. For calcium, the valence is 2, and the atomic mass is 40. Therefore, the equation then becomes (9.0 mg/dL x 10 dL/L x 2) / 40 = 4.5 mEq/L.

Conversion Chart of Metric to English

	Metrix	English
Distance	meter	3.3 feet
Weight	gram	0.0022 pounds
Volume	liter	1.06 quarts

Roman Numerals

The following Roman numerals equal the Arabic numbers.

I = 1
V = 5
X = 10

L = 50
C = 100
D = 500
M = 1000

Military and Civilian Time

Military	=	Civilian
0001	=	12:01 AM
0100	=	1:00 AM
0200	=	2:00 AM
0300	=	3:00 AM
0400	=	4:00 AM
0500	=	5:00 AM
0600	=	6:00 AM
0700	=	7:00 AM
0800	=	8:00 AM
0900	=	9:00 AM
1000	=	10:00 AM
1100	=	11:00 AM
1200	=	12 Noon

Military	=	Civilian
1200	=	12 Noon
1300	=	1:00 PM
1400	=	2:00 PM
1500	=	3:00 PM
1600	=	4:00 PM
1700	=	5:00 PM
1800	=	6:00 PM
1900	=	7:00 PM
2000	=	8:00 PM
2100	=	9:00 PM
2200	=	10:00 PM
2300	=	11:00 PM
0000	=	12 Midnight

Equations to Change Fahrenheit to Celsius and Celsius to Fahrenheit

Fahrenheit into Celsius

$$C = (F - 32) \times 5/9$$

Celsius into Fahrenheit

$$F = (C \times 9/5) + 32$$

Formula to Convert Pounds into Kilograms

$$Kilograms = (Pounds \times 0.4536)$$

Equation to Determine Percentage

$$(amount \div total) \times 100 = percentage$$

Dilution of 1:100 in a Blood Culture Dilution

The dilution of 1:100 means that there is 1mL of blood and 99mL of media for every 100 mL of blood culture specimen.

Approximating Liters of Blood in Normal Adults

The average adult has 70 mL of blood per kilogram of weight. In the United States, a person weigh is usually recorded in pounds. You will need to convert the pounds into kilograms by using the conversion factor of 0.454. The person's weight in kilograms is multiplied by 70 which is the average mL of blood per kilogram. Then divide that number by 1000 to convert the mL into Liters.

Approximating Liters of Blood in Infants

The average infant has 100 mL of blood per kilogram of weight. If an infant's weight is given in pounds it must be converted to kilograms using the conversion factor of 0.454. That number is then multiplied by 100 which is the average mL of blood per kilogram in an infant. Then divide that number by 1000 to convert the mL into liters.

Biological/Biohazardous and Hazardous Waste

Biological wastes are those that contain or are contaminated with pathogens (human, plant, animal); rDNA; and blood, cell, or tissue products; and cultures. Biological wastes that are, or may, be infectious or rDNA contaminated (biohazardous waste) must be inactivated before disposal in hazardous waste containers. Typically, inactivation is carried out with autoclaving or treating with hypochlorite solution (bleach). Contaminated sharps must be maintained in special sharps containers to avoid injury to handlers, and inactivated before disposal. Non-infectious biological wastes, such as uncontaminated gloves, do not require deactivation and are disposed of in biological waste containers. **Hazardous wastes**, those that are ignitable, corrosive, reactive, or toxic, are any that are harmful to humans or the environment and may be solids, liquids, solid gases, or sludges. Hazardous wastes are generally transported by hazardous waste transporters in special hazardous waste containers to Treatment Storage and Disposal Facilities (TSDFs) where they are stored, inactivated, and/or recycled.

Biohazard Symbol

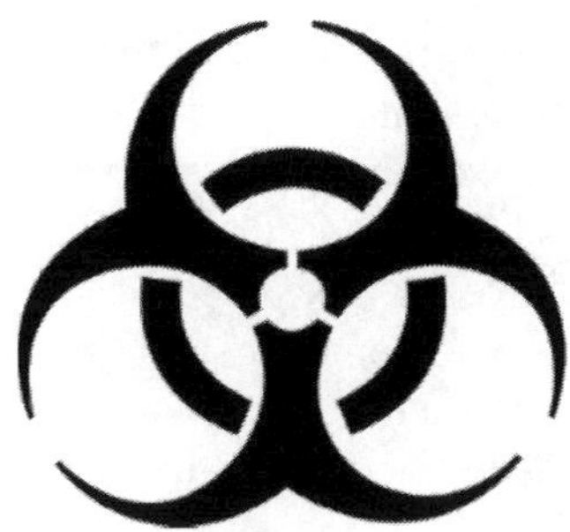

Infection Control Methods

The first line of defense in infection control is hand washing. Protective Clothing is an important aspect of infection control. This includes Masks, Goggles, Face Shields, Respirators, Gowns, Lab Coats, and Gloves. The precautions that are used depend on the infection. Isolation procedures are also used this includes protective isolation or reverse isolation. In protective isolation, the patients are isolated to prevent them from getting an infection i.e. patients receiving chemotherapy. In reverse isolation, the patients are isolated to prevent others from getting their infection or disease i.e. patients with tuberculosis. Universal Precautions are used with all patients. This means do not touch or use anything that has the patient's body fluid on it without a barrier and assume that all body fluid of a patient is infectious.

Chain of Infection

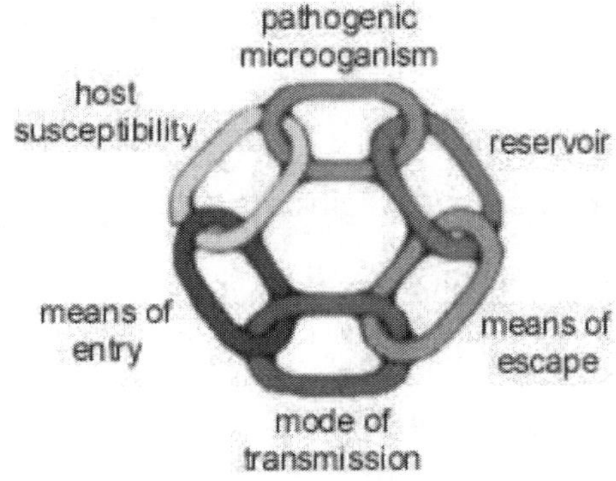

Routes Biological Hazards May Take to Enter the Body

The following are the routes that biological hazards may take to enter the body:

- Airborne (through the nasal passage into the lungs)
- Ingestion (by eating)
- Broken Skin
- Percutaneous (through intact skin)
- Mucosal (through the lining of the mouth and nose)

Hepatitis B

Hepatitis B is explained below:

- Sexually transmitted disease, also transmitted with body fluids and some individual may be symptom free but still be carriers.
- Condoms are not proved to prevent the spread of this disease.
- Symptoms: Jaundice, Dark Urine, Malaise, Joint pain, Fever, Fatigue
- Tests: Decreased albumin levels, + antibodies and antigen, Increased levels of transaminase
- Treatment: Monitor for changes in the liver. Recombinant alpha interferon in some cases. Transplant necessary if liver failure occurs.
- Prevention: Series of 3 Hepatitis B Vaccinations: an initial dose, a dose 1 month later and a final dose 6 months after the initial dose.
- HBV is the most common laboratory-associated infection.

Hepatitis D

Hepatitis D is explained below:

- Usually acquired with HBV as a co-infection or super infection
- Signs and Symptoms: jaundice, fatigue, abdominal pain, loss of appetite, nausea, vomiting, joint pain, dark (tea colored) urine
- Transmission: Occurs when blood from an infected person enters the body of a person who is not immune. By sharing drugs, needles, or "works" when "shooting" drugs; through needle sticks or sharps exposures on the job; or from an infected mother to her baby during birth.
- Treatment: Acute HDV infection - Supportive care. Chronic HDV infection interferon-alfa, liver transplant.
- Prevention: Hepatitis B vaccination, HBV-HDV co-infection - pre- or post-exposure prophylaxis (hepatitis B immune globulin or vaccine) to prevent HBV infection
- HBV-HDV superinfection - education to reduce risk behaviors among persons with chronic HBV infection

Transmission of HIV

The following are ways that HIV can be transmitted from an infected person to an uninfected one:

- Unprotected sexual contact. Direct blood contact, including injection drug needles, blood transfusions, accidents in health care settings or certain blood products. Mother to baby (before or during birth, or through breast milk)
- Sexual intercourse (vaginal and anal): In the genitals and the rectum, HIV may infect the mucous membranes directly or enter through cuts and sores caused during intercourse (many of which would be unnoticed).

- Oral sex (mouth-penis, mouth-vagina): The mouth is an inhospitable environment for HIV (in semen, vaginal fluid or blood), meaning the risk of HIV transmission through the throat, gums, and oral membranes is lower than through vaginal or anal membranes. There are however, documented cases where HIV was transmitted orally.
- Sharing injection needles: An injection needle can pass blood directly from one person's bloodstream to another. It is a very efficient way to transmit a blood-borne virus.
- Mother to Child: It is possible for an HIV-infected mother to pass the virus directly before or during birth, or through breast milk. The following "bodily fluids" are NOT infectious: Saliva, Tears, Sweat, Feces, Urine

Direct and Indirect Contact Transmission

According to the CDC, **contact transmission** is the most common form of disease transmission. Organisms commonly spread through contact include herpes simplex, *Clostridium difficile,* and *Staphylococcus aureus.* Types of contact transmission:

- Direct contact: Transmission is directly from one person to another, usually because of touch. Examples include a person's blood or other body fluids entering broken skin, mucous membranes, or cuts of another person (such as with HIV) and mites (such as scabies) from one person transferring to the another's skin.
- Indirect contact: Transmission occurs from one person, through an intermediary object or person, and then to another person. Examples include when a caregiver's hands touch a patient or bedrails contaminated with a pathogen and then pass that pathogen to a third person (such as with *Clostridium difficile*) and when patient care devices or other items are shared among different patients.

Protocol for Needlestick Injury

If the phlebotomist experiences a **needlestick injury** after carrying out a venipuncture, the phlebotomist's initial response should be to wash the wound with soap and water. As soon as possible, the incident must be reported to a supervisor and steps taken according to established protocol. This may include testing and/or prophylaxis, depending on the patient's health history. In some cases, the patient may also be tested for communicable diseases, such as HIV, in order to determine the risk to the phlebotomist. PEP (post-exposure prophylaxis) is available for exposure to HIV (human immunodeficiency virus) and HBV (hepatitis B virus). However, no PEP is available for HCV (hepatitis C virus) although the CDC does provide a plan for management. PEP should be initiated within 72 hours of exposure. All testing and treatments associated with the needlestick injury must be provided free of cost to the phlebotomist.

Putting on and Removing Protective Clothing

A healthcare worker puts on the protective gown first being sure not to touch the outside of the gown. The mask in put on next. Gloves are applied last and secured over the cuffs of the gown. A healthcare worker removes the gloves first. They are removed by grasping one glove at the wrist and pulling it inside out off the hand and holding it in the gloved hand. The second glove is removed by placing your uncovered hands fingers under the edge of the glove being careful not to touch the outside of the glove and rolling it down inside out over the glove grasped in your hand. The first glove ends up inside of the second glove. Next, slide arms out of the gown and then fold the gown with the outside folded in away from the body so that the contaminated side is folded inwardly. Dispose of properly. Finally, remove the mask by touching the strings only. Always wash hands after glove removal.

Cleaning Up Small Blood Spills

The best way to clean a small blood spill is to absorb the blood with a paper towel or gauze pad. Then disinfect area with a disinfectant. Soap and water is not a disinfectant nor is alcohol. Never scrape a dry spill; this may cause an aerosol of infectious organisms. If blood is dried, use the disinfectant to moisten the dried blood.

General Knowledge of Fire Safety

Fire requires three components to occur. They are called the fire triangle and include fuel, oxygen, and heat when a chemical source is included it forms the fire tetrahedron. In the event of a fire remember these two acronyms, RACE and PASS. RACE describes the steps for dealing with a fire. "R" stands for Rescue (rescue patients and co-workers from danger.) "A" stands for alarm (sound the alarm and alert those around you.) "C" stands for confine (confine a fire by closing the doors and windows.) "E" stands for extinguish (use the nearest fire extinguisher to put out the fire. PASS describes how to use a fire extinguisher to put out a fire. "P" stands for pull the pin. "A" stands for aim at the fire. "S" stands for squeeze the trigger. "S" stands for sweep the base of the fire. Fires are broken down into four classes. Class A fires involve ordinary combustible materials. Class B fires involve flammable liquids, Class C involves electrical fires, and Class D involves combustible metals.

Patient Consents

The types of patient consents needed to do a procedure are as follows:

- Informed Consent - a competent person gives voluntary permission for a medical procedure after receiving adequate information about the risk of, methods used and consequences of the procedure
- Expressed Consent - permission given by patient verbally or in writing for a procedure
- Implied Consent - the patient's actions gives permission for the procedure without verbal or written consent for example going to the emergency room or holding out arm when told need to draw blood.
- HIV Consent - special permission given to administer a test for detecting the human immunodeficiency virus.
- Parental Consent for Minors - a parent or a legal guardian must give permission for procedures administered to underage patients depending on the state law may range from 18 to 21 years old.

POA MS-DRG

On admission to acute hospitals under the Medicare Inpatient Prospective Payment System (IPPS), patients must be given a **present-on-admission (POA)** Medicare Severity Diagnosis Related Group (MS-DRG) diagnosis. The MS-DRG should include primary and secondary diagnoses present during the admission process. This is a concern regarding maximizing reimbursement because hospital-acquired conditions may not be covered if there is a change at discharge from the POA diagnosis. A POA indicator must be on all claims:

- Y: Medicare pays for condition if HAC present and accounted for on admission.
- N: Medicare will not pay for condition if HAC is present on discharge but not on admission.
- U: Medicare will not pay for condition if HAC is present and documentation is not adequate to determine if the condition was present on admission.
- W: Medicare will pay for condition if HAC is present and the healthcare provider cannot determine if the condition was present on admission.

LIABILITY

Liability is legal responsibility for something the individual has done or failed to do. Element of liability include:

- Neglect: Failure to provide basic needs or usual standards or care or exhibiting of uncaring attitude toward a patient.
- Abandonment: A unilateral severing of the professional relationship between the healthcare provider and the patient with no notice that would allow the patient to make other arrangements.
- Assault: A threat to touch another person against the patient's will, such as threatening to withdraw blood from an uncooperative patient.
- Battery: Following through with a threat and touching another person without consent, such as forcing the patient to undergo venipuncture.
- Tort: Negligent act that causes injury or suffering to another person and is the basis for a civil action, such as a lawsuit.
- Malpractice: Failure to meet standards of care or wrongfully carrying out duties in such a way as to bring harm to a patient.

HIPAA AND CONFIDENTIALITY

The **Health Insurance Portability and Accountability Act** (HIPAA) addresses the rights of the individual related to confidentiality of health information. Healthcare providers must not release any information or documentation about a patient's condition or treatment without consent, as the individual has the right to determine who has access to personal information. Personal information about the patient is considered protected health information (PHI), and consists of any identifying or personal information about the patient, such as health history, condition, or treatments in any form, and any documentation, including electronic, verbal, or written. Personal information can be shared with a spouse, legal guardians, those with durable power of attorney for the patient, and those involved in care of the patient, such as physicians, without a specific release, but the patient should always be consulted if personal information is to be discussed with others present to ensure there is no objection. Failure to comply with HIPAA regulations can make one liable for legal action.

AMERICANS WITH DISABILITIES ACT

The 1990 **Americans with Disabilities Act (ADA)** is civil rights legislation that provides the disabled, including those with mental impairment, access to employment and the community. The ADA covers not only obvious disabilities but also disorders such as arthritis, seizure disorders, cardiovascular and respiratory disorders. Communities must provide transportation services for the disabled, including accommodation for wheelchairs. Public facilities (schools, museums, physician's offices, post offices, restaurants, hospitals, laboratories) must be accessible with ramps and elevators as needed. Telecommunications must also be accessible through devices or accommodations for the deaf and blind. Laboratories must accommodate those with disabilities and may need to provide sign language translators or other methods of communicating with patients when necessary. Some patients, such as those who are legally blind, may have service animals (only a dog), and these animals must be allowed to accompany the person in all public areas. Comfort animals are not covered by the ADA.

SCOPE OF PRACTICE AND ETHICAL STANDARDS RELATED TO PRACTICE OF PHLEBOTOMY

The **scope of practice** encompasses those duties and procedures that the person's training, licensure and/or certification, has prepared the person to undertake. The phlebotomist and other laboratory professionals must adhere to the **code of ethics** developed by the American Society for Clinical Laboratory Sciences (ASCLS):

- Duty to patient: This is the primary focus and depends on being honest, showing respect for the patient, and providing a high standard of care
- Duty to colleagues and profession: The phlebotomist and laboratory professionals must establish an honest and cooperative working relationship with colleagues and work to improve personal practice and to advance the profession,
- Duty to society: The phlebotomist and laboratory professionals must comply with laws and regulations and serve as patient advocates.
- Pledge: The phlebotomist and laboratory professionals pledge to carry out the duties outlines in the code of ethics, beginning with placing the welfare of the patient before that of self.

Deming's 14 Points for Quality Improvement

Deming's 14 points:

1. Create and communicate to all employees a statement of the quality philosophy of the company.
2. Adopt this philosophy.
3. Build quality into a product throughout production.
4. End the practice of awarding business on the basis of price tag alone; build a long-term relationship based on established loyalty and trust.
5. Work to constantly improve quality and productivity.
6. Institute on-the-job quality training.
7. Teach and institute leadership to improve all job functions.
8. Drive out fear; create trust.
9. Strive to reduce inter- and intradepartmental conflicts.
10. Eliminate slogans and targets; instead, focus on the system and morale.
11. Eliminate numerical quotas for production and management. Substitute leadership methods for improvement.
12. Remove barriers that rob people of pride in their work.
13. Educate with self-improvement programs.
14. Include everyone in the company to accomplish the transformation.

Role of Laboratory Professional in Customer Service/Support

All laboratory professionals serve a role in **customer service and support** to some degree because they represent the organization with every patient contact, and the patient's attitude toward the organization may be based on this contact. The three components in any delivery of service are the customer (patient, family member, visitor), the organization (laboratory, hospitals), and the individual service provider (lab professional). For this reason, it's important that the individual remain professional, showing respect and consideration for the patient and others, maintaining a professional appearance, and carrying out duties competently. Communication is the essential element in customer service, including both conveying information in language appropriate to the listener and being an active listener. The laboratory professional should try to anticipate patient concerns, provide reassurance, and answer any questions in a positive straightforward manner. Body language and words should both convey sincerity, and the laboratory professional should always handle complaints in a positive manner.

Medicare Health Plans

Medicare Health Plans include are managed care plans such as Medicare Advantage organizations, cost plans, or health care prepayment plans. Services provided by contract providers (those who participate in these plans) are reimbursed by Medicare. However, non-contract providers (those outside of these plans who provide services to enrollees (patients), such a laboratory) may not be reimbursed. If Medicare denies payment to a non-contract provider, that provider must receive notice regarding the reason for the denial and steps to appeal the decision. The filing for reconsideration must be done within 60 days from the date of notification and must include a signed Waiver of Liability form. The form contains the enrollees Medicare number and name, the name of the non-contract provider, the dates of service, and the name of the health plan. The waiver of liability statement waives any right to collect payment for the services provided regardless of the outcome of the appeal process although the provider maintains the right to further appeal.

Written Orders for Tests

Written and signed orders must be received for all tests, so telephone orders or verbal orders (such as in emergency situations) must be followed by a signed written order, which can be delivered, mailed, or electronically submitted to the laboratory. Tests may be ordered by the physician, the advanced practice nurse (such as a nurse practitioner,) or physician's assistant caring for the patient. The ordering healthcare provider must document in the patient's record the intention of having the test performed and the medical necessity for the test. Written orders should contain the date ordered, the time the test should be carried out, and diagnostic code (ICD-10-CM) for each test ordered. The order should be appropriate for the diagnostic code, or CMS and insurance companies may not reimburse for the cost of the test.

Reporting and Documenting Abnormal and Critical Laboratory Test Results

Abnormal laboratory test results are those that are outside of normal values:

- Abnormal: These results are not considered urgent or critical although the laboratory report should be transmitted to the ordering healthcare provider as soon as possible. For example, a fasting glucose of 108 is slightly elevated but does not generally pose an immediate risk to the patient. Reports may be reported by various means: verbal, telephone, electronic. In all cases, the receiver must acknowledge receipt of the laboratory results.
- Critical required: These are tests that must be completed for a specific purpose and by a specific time, so all test results (whether abnormal or not) should be immediately reported. Must be reported through direct communication (verbal, telephone, or hand-delivered). If per telephone, the receiver must repeat back the lab results.
- Critical: These results point to a condition that may be life-threatening if not immediately attended to, such as an elevated potassium level. Must also be reported through direct communication as above.

The time and date that the lab reports were delivered, the receiver, and the acknowledgement must be documented.

Proper Telephone Technique and Etiquette

Laboratory professionals often must answer the **telephone** or make calls, such as to verify orders or report orders. When taking calls, the individual should answer with the name of the laboratory and personal name, "Hello, this is Smith Laboratory, J. Doe speaking. How can I help you?" For receiving and reporting orders, a script should be prepared and followed (not necessarily word for word) to ensure that all necessary information is received and conveyed. The laboratory professional should know how to answer the phone, how to put a caller on hold, and how to transfer calls as needed. Additionally, prioritizing calls is essential if calls are frequent and some may need to be put on hold. Callers should always be asked before being placed on hold. When taking calls, the laboratory professional should have a pen and paper available to take notes as needed. The laboratory professional should remain calm and supportive, trying to diffuse any angry calls: "I'm sorry you're upset. I do understand and will try to help you."

Charting or Filing Reports Properly

Documenting and filing reports varies according to the type of records the organization uses. With paper records, the laboratory report is sent to the correct nursing station, department, or office through pneumatic tube, hand delivery, or courier. If placing the report directly, the laboratory professional should verify the patient's name and ID number to ensure the record is placed in the correct patient record and in the correct section of the record, generally with the latest reports first. If filing electronically, in some cases the reports will be filed in the patient's electronic health record automatically according to the patient's assigned barcode. If entered manually into the electronic health record, the patient's name and ID number must, as with paper records, be verified. Health records are set up and managed in different ways, so the procedures in place for each system must be followed.

Equipment in the Hospital Environment

Equipment used in the hospital environment includes:

- Pager (beeper): Low cost device that signals the user. Can be used to send encrypted digital or voice messages although communication is unidirectional. Often used to notify laboratory professionals of new orders.
- Automated menu (telephone): Usually refers to telephone menus that give the caller options, such as "press one for admissions and records." Options should be limited to 2 to 5 and levels to no more than 2 or callers will likely hang up. One choice for callers should be to speak to an operator.
- Switchboard: Telecommunication system used to correctly route telephone calls through a system, such as to different departments or individuals (patients, staff members).
- Photocopier: Machine that copies paper documents, such as to provide patients with copies of their records. They usually include scanning capability and may, for example, be used to scan and copy patient's Medicare and insurance cards.
- Fax (facsimile): Allows paper documents to be scanned and sent through telephone lines to another party, where the receiving fax machine prints a copy. Frequently used to transmit laboratory or other reports.

Propriety and Professionalism

A laboratory professional is expected to demonstrate both **propriety and professionalism** in order to gain respect of other professionals and the public. Propriety is the state of conforming to accepted behavior and moral standards while professionalism is conducting oneself with the competency expected of those in the profession. Elements of propriety and professionalism include:

- Appearance: The individual should be neat and clean and dressed in the appropriate uniform or lab coat. Hair should be neatly combed and nails clean and trimmed. The individual should wear a nametag or badge showing the name and position, such as "Phlebotomist" or "Laboratory technician."
- Conduct: The individual should carry out duties appropriately and honestly and treat others with respect and consideration. The individual should adhere to the code of ethics of the profession in all professional matters.
- Communication: All forms of communication (verbal, digital, telephone, written) should be carried out in a professional manner, avoiding slang, jargon, profanity, and sarcasm. The individual should communicate actions and intentions and listen actively to others.

Doctrine of Respondeat Superior

Respondeat superior is Latin for "let the master answer" and is the basis for the legal doctrine that employers or supervisors are responsible for the acts of their agents/employees. This doctrine makes it illegal for employers to profit from criminal acts of subordinates and also makes them culpable for acts of negligence or malpractice on the part of subordinates (vicarious liability). For this reason, if a medical laboratory technician is negligent, the victim can bring a civil suit against the person in charge of the laboratory and the organization to which the laboratory belongs. Because of this doctrine, it's especially important that a laboratory have clear policies and procedures and adhere to accepted national standards. Employers must be informed about these standards and trained in all policies and procedures and should be effectively supervised.

Nonverbal Communication

Nonverbal communication is involved in most communication, and is usually automatic and is not a conscious process. Nonverbal communication is good for connecting with patients and communicating feelings or mood, but is not useful for communicating specific information. Nonverbal communication can include body language, facial expressions, vocalizations, and eye contact.

- Facial expressions: The face can show numerous emotions, and the words being used should usually match the facial expression. If the voice and face do not match, miscommunication can take place, as the listener may perceive the speaker as ingenuine or lying. Facial expressions should be used to reinforce the intended message and tone.
- Vocal signals: Nonverbal vocal signals refer to sounds made, other than words, such as sighing, saying "mmm-hmm" to communicate tone or mood. The method of delivery of speech, such as pace, pitch, and volume are considered part of verbal communication, but can also indicate and reinforce emotions in conversation.
- Eye contact: Eye contact varies with cultures, and one should follow cultural cues, but for most Americans, there is a line between maintaining eye contact and staring. A good balance includes enough eye contact to communicate attention, but not so much eye contact that it makes someone uncomfortable by communicating intimidation or overconfidence.
- Body language: People may present their bodies with different tones by changing how they stand. An open position, arms to the side or outstretched, and leaning forward suggest trust and care. A closed position, with arms folded, legs crossed, and leaning backwards can serve as a barrier to conversation. Body language is helpful, but unreliable by itself. A closed position can indicate pain, feeling cold, unwillingness, or mistrust. An open position can be used to help connect and build trust between a professional and their client. Leaning toward a person when speaking shows interest and helps to put the other person at ease.
- Gestures: Hand gestures can be used to signify understanding or confusion, to accentuate a point, to indicate directions, or pantomime an activity. People often nod their heads in agreement or disagreement.
- Personal Space: The personal space and distance between people at which people feel comfortable varies by culture, and the laboratory professional should observe and match the distance established by their patients and family. For communication in a professional space, a healthy distance of four to seven feet is generally preferred.

Important Terms

CAP: College of American Pathologists offers the Laboratory Accreditation Program (LAP), which accredits all types of laboratories, including those in hospitals and physician's office.

COLA: Commission on Laboratory Accreditation, was founded in 1988 with the original intent of inspecting and accrediting physician office laboratories to ensure that they were in compliance with CLIA (Clinical Laboratory Improvement Amendments). COLA has since expanded its mission and now also accredits hospital laboratories as well as independent laboratories. CMS (Center for Medicare and Medicaid) and TJC (Joint Commission) have granted deeming authority to COLA.

AABB: The American Association of Blood Banks sets standards for blood collection as well as processing, testing, distributing and administering blood/blood products and accredits facilities that carry out these functions.

Tort: An injury or wrong committed, either with or without force, to the person or property of another, for which civil liability may be imposed.

Assault: The touching of another person with an intent to harm, without that person's consent, A willful attempt to illegally inflict injury on or threaten a person

Malpractice: A lawsuit raised against a professional for injury or loss resulting from negligence on the part of the professional in rendering services.

Negligence: Failure to perform or act with the prudence expected by a reasonable person in the same circumstance.

Vicarious liability: When a person is held responsible for the tort of another even though the person being held responsible may not have done anything wrong. This is often the case with employers who are held vicariously liable for the damages caused by their employees.

Breach of confidentiality: Occurs when information that should be kept secret, with access limited to appropriate persons, is given to an inappropriate person

Fraud: An intentional perversion of truth; deceitful practice or device resorted to with intent to deprive another of property or other right.

Gram: Basic metric unit of weight

Meter: Basic metric unit of distance

Liter: Basic metric unit of volume

Communicable Infection: An illness caused by the direct or indirect transmission of a specific infectious agent or the toxins it produces from an infected person, animal, or inanimate host to a susceptible body; indirect transmission can be via a vector, intermediate plant or animal host, or the inanimate environment.

Nosocomial Infection: Hospital-acquired illness not resulting from the original reason for the patient to be admitted.

MLA Practice Test

1. Receiving cannot accept a specimen unless it has:

a. A correct, legible label
b. An uncontaminated, signed requisition with billing information
c. An intact container with correct media
d. All of the above

2. A laboratory refrigerator used to store volatile, flammable liquids can hold:

a. 120 gallons of class I, II, and IIIA liquids
b. 180 gallons of class I, II, and IIIA liquids
c. 200 gallons of class I, II, and IIIA liquids
d. 50 gallons of class I, II, and IIIA liquids

3. Disease incidence predicts:

a. How probable it is a patient will develop a disease, and its etiology
b. How likely a test result is to be right or wrong, given certain variables
c. How likely the patient with a negative test really does not have the condition
d. How likely the patient with a positive test result really has the condition

4. Beer's law in spectrophotometry

a. Means a transparent sample transmits 0% light
b. Only applies if absorbance is between 0.1 and 1.0
c. Means an opaque sample transmits 100% light
d. Uses a visible spectrum from 340 nm to 500 nm

5. Naming bacteria by looking at their size and shape under the microscope, and the colony morphology on media is:

a. Differential identification
b. Numeric taxonomy
c. Presumptive identification
d. TaqMan electrophoresis

6. The hospital department that studies alcohol, drugs, poisons, and heavy metals is:

a. Serology/Immunology
b. Toxicology
c. Cytology
d. Endocrinology

7. A hemoglobin electrophoresis result of adult hemoglobin (HbA) or HbA2 means the patient has:

a. Sickle cell anemia
b. Fetal hemoglobin
c. Normal hemoglobin
d. Hemolytic anemia

8. The recall rate is also known as the:

a. Sensitivity
b. Specificity
c. Aliquot
d. Circadian rhythm

9. Biochemistry usually requires:

a. Lavender, light blue, and black blood collection tubes
b. Red, pink, and yellow blood collection tubes
c. Green, gray, and marbled serum-separator tube (SST) blood collection tubes
d. Navy, purple, and brown blood collection tubes

10. A normal kidney function study shows a:

a. BUN to creatinine ratio between 15:1 and 20:1
b. Alkaline phosphatase 30 to 85 international milliunits/mL
c. Serum aspartate aminotransferase 5 to 40 international units/L
d. Amylase 56 to 190 international units/L

11. A newborn's jaundice could be caused by:

a. Erythroblastosis fetalis
b. Kernicterus
c. Physiologic jaundice from poor fluid intake
d. All of the above

12. Lipids from carbohydrate and alcohol sources are:

a. Anions
b. Triglycerides
c. Cholesterol
d. Eluent

13. When serum protein indicates disease, the doctor usually follows up with:

a. Total protein, albumin, and globulin
b. Ascites
c. Protein electrophoresis
d. Bilirubin

14. Elevated creatine phosphokinase (CPK) could mean myocardial infarction, but could also mean:

a. Alcoholism, hypothyroidism, cardioversion, or clofibrate use
b. Aspirin, burns, warfarin, or sickle cell anemia
c. Lung disease or congestive heart failure
d. Crushing injury, bowel infarction, or opiate use

15. A patient whose cortisol level is high at both 8:00 a.m. and 4:00 p.m. likely has:

a. Addison's disease
b. Natriuretic factor
c. Diabetes insipidus
d. Cushing syndrome

16. Decreased sodium in the blood is:

a. Hypernatremia, often from diabetes, burns, or Cushing syndrome
b. Hyponatremia, often from vomiting and diarrhea, furosemide, or Addison's disease
c. Hyperkalemia, often from acidosis, spironolactone, or kidney failure
d. Hypokalemia, often from alkalosis, stomach cancer, or eating too much licorice

17. CPK in a patient with a myocardial infarction will:

a. Rise 6 hours after heart attack, peak in 18 hours, and return to baseline in 3 days
b. Rise 6 to 10 hours after heart attack, peak at 12 to 48 hours, and return to baseline in 4 days
c. Rise 24 to 72 hours after heart attack, peak in 4 days, and return to baseline in 14 days
d. Cause a corresponding rise in alpha-fetoprotein

18. The liver destroys old blood cells at the end of their lifespan of:

a. 120 days
b. 30 days
c. 1 week
d. 90 days

19. An erythrocyte sedimentation rate (ESR) measures how blood cells with anticoagulant aggregate in a Westergren or Wintrobe tube in 1 hour because of changes in plasma proteins, which is known as :

a. Retic count
b. Serendipity
c. Fibrinolysis
d. Rouleaux formation

20. If the doctor suspects the patient has Hodgkin's disease, then the correct stain for the smear is:

a. Periodic acid-Schiff (PAS)
b. Sudan black B (SBB)
c. Leukocyte alkaline phosphatase (LAP)
d. Lactophenol cotton blue (LPCB)

21. A battlement scan is preferable to a wedge scan for studying bone marrow because:

a. Battlement technique distributes cells evenly across the slide
b. Lymphocytes concentrate in the feather
c. Wedge technique causes leukocytes to pool in different sections of the slide
d. Both a and c

22. Most coagulation (clotting) disorders are due to:

a. Phase I problems
b. Factor VIII deficiency
c. Fibrinolysis
d. Factor III distress call from the injury site

23. If the patient's PT and PTT are longer than 70 seconds, then check if ______ caused a false result:

a. Ferritin
b. Lupus inhibitor antibody (LA)
c. Platelet antibody
d. Intrinsic factor

24. Confirm a fungal infection found through microscopy with a:

a. Latex serology for cryptococcal antigen
b. Fungal serology titer of more than 1:32 that increases x4 or more 3 weeks later
c. Complement fixation for coccidiomycosis and histoplasmosis
d. Immunodiffusion for blastomycosis.

25. Two modern flocculation tests that replace the older Venereal Disease Research Laboratory (VDRL) test for syphilis screening are:

a. Plasmacrit test (PCT) and rapid plasma reagin (RPR) test
b. Fluorescent treponemal antibody absorption (FTA-ABS) and enzyme-linked immunosorbent assay (ELISA)
c. Treponemal-specific microhemagglutination (MHA-TP) and T. pallidum particle agglutination test (TP-PA)
d. Captia Syphilis-G enzyme immunoassay (EIA) and cold agglutinins

26. To make a dilution of ½ or 1:2

a. Dilute ½ ml of serum with 2 mL of saline
b. Dilute 1 ml of serum with 2 mL of saline
c. Test undiluted serum for antibody/antigen reaction against a control
d. Dilute 1 mL of serum with 1 mL of saline

27. A Monospot test uses ingredients from:

a. Guinea pig, cow, and horse
b. Sheep, pig, and horse
c. Dog, sheep, and rabbit
d. Fish, cat, and ferret

28. A prozone phenomenon occurs when performing an antibody titer on a patient with:

a. Epstein-Barr virus (EBV)
b. Reynaud disease
c. Both syphilis and HIV
d. Immunoglobulin G (IgG) antibodies

29. An Rh- mother who is pregnant with the child of an Rh+ father needs Rh immunoglobulin (RhoGAM):

a. Even if the pregnancy ends in miscarriage or abortion
b. At 26 to 28 weeks of pregnancy and again within 72 hours after her delivery.
c. During her labor
d. Both a and b

30. If your patient has a mild transfusion reaction:

a. Eosinophilia, hypocalcemia, leukopenia, and pancytopenia may occur
b. Dyscrasia, leukocytosis, hypercalcemia, and leukemia may occur
c. Anemia, hypokalemia, glycosuria, and pancytopenia may occur
d. Hemolysis, hyperkalemia, hypoglycemia, and hemoglobinuria may occur

31. Type O blood has:

a. B antigen and anti-A antibody
b. A antigen and anti-B antibody
c. No A or B antigens and both anti-A and anti-B antibodies
d. Both A and B antigens and no anti-A or anti-B antibodies

32. Choose the top priority transfusion patient from the list below.

a. Cardiac surgery patient who lost more than 1,200 mL of blood
b. Trauma patient with a hemoglobin of 5 g/dL
c. Pernicious anemia patient
d. Hemophiliac boy at regular clinic visit

33. Reject a transfusion request when:

a. Recipient blood specimen is hemolyzed
b. The patient armband does not have a unique identifier
c. Donor blood is lipemic, clotted, or contains foreign objects
d. All of the above

34. To diagnose a urinary tract infection correctly, the microbiology lab requires a:

a. Midstream urine collection (MSU)
b. Witnessed urine collection
c. 24-hour urine collection
d. Random urine collection

35. When assisting the doctor with cerebrospinal fluid (CSF) collection, you need 4 tubes for:

a. Cell count, glucose and protein, gram stain and culture, virology/mycology/cytology.
b. Immunoelectrophoresis
c. Fungus, oncology, and SMA-12
d. Neutrophilia, lymphocytophilia, glutamine, and lactate dehydrogenase (LDH)

36. Fusobacteria cause:

a. Botulism and Listeria infections
b. Lyme disease and Helicobacter pylori stomach ulcers
c. Pyorrhea and Lemierre syndrome
d. Chlamydia genital infections and pneumonia

37. The type of media required to incubate a TB culture correctly is:

a. Tinsdale
b. Sheep blood agar
c. Modified Wadowsky-Yee (MWY)
d. Löwenstein-Jensen (LJ) egg

38. To find parasites under the microscope, set the magnification to:

a. 40x
b. 10x
c. 1000x
d. 400x

39. Identify the parasite that must be reported to Public Health authorities:

a. Crypto (Cryptosporidium parvum)
b. Hookworm (Ancylostoma duodenale)
c. Tapeworm (Cestoda)
d. Pinworm (Enterobius)

40. To identify motile trophozoites:

a. Examine blood smears and blood antigens
b. Perform a string test
c. Use Snap n' Stain on sputum
d. Wet mount fresh, liquid stool with LPCB stain

41. Public Health requires you to keep positive parasitology samples preserved for :

a. The patient's lifetime
b. One year
c. Ten years
d. One month

42. Shine a Wood's lamp over the patient's skin to help you collect:

a. Malaria specimens
b. Public Health specimens
c. Toxicology specimens
d. Mycology specimens

43. Identify the positive dipstick test that would indicate an E. coli infection:

a. Leukocytes
b. Protein
c. Ketones
d. Nitrites

44. A pregnancy test may be ordered for a man with:

a. Testicular cancer
b. Prostatitis
c. Cryptorchidism
d. Peyronie disease

45. Normal urinary output for a 24-hour urine test is:

a. 4 quarts
b. 150 to 500 mL
c. 30 liters
d. 750 to 2,000 mL

46. Urate crystals found during microscopic urinalysis indicate:

a. Urea-splitting bacteria are present
b. Poisoning
c. Gout
d. Hyperparathyroidism

47. Patients with polycystic kidney disease (PKD) often have:

a. Cirrhosis and hepatitis
b. Coronary artery bypass graft (CABG) and hypertension
c. Hematuria and uroliths
d. Melena and hematochezia

48. Transfer of an infectious agent via droplets larger than 5 μm in diameter is known as

a. Airborne transmission
b. Droplet transmission
c. Vector transmission
d. Vehicle transmission

49. Which of the following is an example of vector transmission?

a. Tuberculosis
b. Salmonella infection
c. Bubonic plague
d. HIV

50. Droplet transmission may result from

a. Mosquito bite
b. Kissing
c. Contaminated food or water
d. Throat swab

51. All of the following are prohibited under Centers for Disease Control (CDC) guidelines for hand hygiene EXCEPT

a. Hand washing using plain soap and water
b. Artificial nails
c. Nails longer than one quarter inch
d. Touching faucet handles after hand washing

52. Protective isolation may be required for all of the following patients EXCEPT

a. Neutropenic chemotherapy patients
b. Burn patients
c. Infants
d. AIDS patients

53. Which of the following statements regarding standard precautions for infection control is FALSE?

a. Use both hands to recap needles
b. Hands should be washed before putting on and after removing gloves
c. Standard precautions apply to all secretions except sweat
d. Resuscitation devices may be used as an alternative to the mouth-to-mouth method

54. Use of an N95 respirator is NOT required in the case of

a. A child with chickenpox
b. A child with measles
c. An adult immune to measles or chickenpox
d. An adult who has never had measles or chickenpox

55. Which of the following is NOT a violation of general laboratory safety rules?

a. Wearing a laboratory coat when leaving the lab
b. Wearing nail polish
c. Wearing large earrings
d. Having shoulder-length hair

56. Which of the following statements regarding HBV is FALSE?

a. HBV vaccine also protects against HDV
b. HBV vaccine does not contain live virus
c. HBV vaccine may pose a risk of HBV transmission
d. HBV can survive up to 1 week in dried blood

57. HCV exposure may occur through

a. Urine
b. Sexual contact
c. Semen
d. Phlebotomy procedures

58. To reduce the risk of transmission of a bloodborne pathogen, you should

a. Cleanse the wound with bleach
b. Cleanse the wound with an antiseptic
c. Cleanse the wound with soap and water
d. Squeeze the wound to release fluid

59. A specific type of fire extinguisher is used for each of the following classes of fire EXCEPT

a. Class K
b. Class D
c. Class C
d. Class B

60. A fire caused by the splashing of hot grease from a frying pan is classified as a

a. Class K fire
b. Class A fire
c. Class B fire
d. Class D fire

61. All of the following are acceptable procedures to control wound hemorrhage EXCEPT

a. Applying direct pressure to the wound
b. Using an elastic bandage to hold the compress
c. Removing the original compress when adding additional material
d. Using cloth or gauze to apply pressure

62. Which of the following symbols is NOT included on the Joint Commission "Do Not Use" list?

a. IU
b. IV
c. U
d. QD

63. A patient lying on their stomach is said to be in the

a. Anatomic position
b. Prone position
c. Supine position
d. Reclining position

64. Which of the following statements regarding lumbar puncture is FALSE?

a. The needle enters the spinal cavity
b. The needle enters the space between the 3rd and 4th lumbar vertebrae
c. The procedure poses a risk of injury to the spinal cord
d. The procedure does not present a risk of spinal cord injury

65. The hormone epinephrine

a. Increases blood pressure and heart rate
b. Controls thyroid activity
c. Is associated with SAD
d. Decreases urine production

66. Increased levels of which of the following are associated with heart attack?

a. Albumin
b. PSA
c. CK
d. CEA

67. Which of the following is the recommended order of draw for syringes?

a. The SST follows the red top
b. The red top follows the SST
c. The gray top is first
d. Sterile specimens are last

68. According to the alternate order of draw for syringes,

a. The light-blue top is first
b. The lavender top is first
c. The red top and SST are last
d. The gray top is last

69. A sign with a picture of fall leaves may be used to indicate

a. Do not resuscitate order
b. Miscarriage
c. No blood pressures in right arm
d. Fall precautions

70. Which of the following statements regarding obtaining a blood specimen from a patient is FALSE?

a. The phlebotomist should ask the patient's permission before collecting blood
b. The patient has the right to refuse blood draw
c. The name of the ordering physician on the ID band should not differ
d. Patient identity should always be verified

71. Which of the following statements regarding patient identification is FALSE?

a. Outpatients may be identified by an ID card
b. Outpatients should be asked to state their name and date of birth
c. If a patient has been identified by the receptionist, no further verification is needed
d. A patient's response when his or her name is called is not sufficient for identification

72. The preferred venipuncture site is the

a. Cephalic vein
b. Median cubital vein
c. Median basilic vein
d. Median cephalic vein

73. All of the following statements regarding tourniquet application are true EXCEPT

a. The patient should be told to pump his fist
b. A tourniquet may be applied over the patient's sleeve
c. Two tourniquets may be used together
d. A tourniquet should not be applied over an open sore

74. If an antecubital vein cannot be located, you may

a. Use a vein on the underside of the wrist
b. Perform a capillary puncture
c. Manipulate the site until a vein can be found
d. Use a tendon

75. Which of the following statements regarding blood specimens is FALSE?

a. Outpatient and inpatient blood specimens have the same normal values
b. Hemoglobin and hematocrit have higher normal ranges at higher elevations
c. Caffeine may affect cortisol levels
d. Ingestion of butter or cheese may produce a milky specimen

76. Blood levels of which of the following are normally lowest during the morning?

a. Iron
b. Insulin
c. Potassium
d. Glucose

77. Exercise increases levels of all of the following EXCEPT

a. Protein
b. Cholesterol
c. Liver enzymes
d. Skeletal muscle enzymes

78. All of the following affect blood specimen composition EXCEPT

a. Body position
b. Temperature and humidity
c. Fasting
d. Stress

79. In which of the following patients is blood collection prohibited?

a. Patient with a hematoma
b. Pregnant patient
c. Mastectomy patient
d. Patient with a tattoo

80. A patient begins to faint during blood collection. The most appropriate line of action would be to

a. Use an ammonia inhalant to revive the patient
b. Continue the draw and quickly withdraw the needle
c. Apply pressure to the site and lower the patient's head
d. Allow the patient to leave after regaining consciousness

81. All of the following may trigger hematoma EXCEPT

a. Small veins
b. Inadequate pressure to the site
c. Needle penetration all the way through the vein
d. Petechiae

82. To prevent hemoconcentration during venipuncture, you should

a. Massage the area until a vein is located
b. Ask the patient to release his or her fist when blood flow begins
c. Ask the patient to vigorously pump his or her fist
d. Redirect the needle several times until a vein is located

83. Hemolysis may result from all of the following EXCEPT

a. Filling the tube until the normal amount of vacuum is exhausted
b. Partially filling a sodium fluoride tube
c. Liver disease
d. Pulling back the plunger too quickly

84. Under which of the following conditions is underfilling additive tubes UNACCEPTABLE?

a. When drawing blood from children
b. When drawing blood from anemic patients
c. When using a red top or SST
d. As a time-saving strategy

85. Which of the following is NOT a cause of vein collapse?

a. Tourniquet too close to the venipuncture site
b. Vacuum draw of the tube
c. Stoppage of blood flow on tourniquet removal
d. Rolling veins

86. Capillary puncture is the preferred method for

a. Dehydrated patients
b. Newborns
c. Coagulation studies
d. Blood cultures

87. The recommended site for capillary puncture is the

a. Tip of the finger
b. Big toe
c. Index finger
d. Middle finger

88. A safe area for capillary puncture in infants is the

a. Medial plantar surface of the heel
b. Posterior curvature of the heel
c. Arch of the foot
d. Earlobe

89. Which of the following statements regarding warming techniques is FALSE?

a. Warming the site is necessary for collecting blood gas specimens
b. Warming is required for fingersticks in patients with cold hands
c. Warming significantly alters results of routine analyte testing
d. Warming is recommended for heelstick procedures in infants

90. Proper blood collection procedure includes

a. Wiping away the first drop of blood
b. Applying strong repetitive pressure on the site
c. Using a scooping motion to collect blood as it flows down the finger
d. Removing the tube from the drop

91. Proper procedure for TB testing includes

a. Applying pressure to the site
b. Wiping the site with gauze
c. Avoiding areas of the arm with excessive hair
d. Applying a bandage to the site

92. Collection timing is most critical for

a. Phenobarbital
b. Digoxin
c. Ethanol
d. Aminoglycosides

93. Which of the following disinfectants may be used for ETOH testing?

a. Tincture of iodine
b. Soap and water
c. Isopropyl alcohol
d. Methanol

94. Abnormal bone function caused by a lack of vitamin D in the diet is known as

a. Arthritis
b. Osteochondritis
c. Rickets
d. Osteomyelitis

95. Which of the following is a form of arthritis?

a. Bursitis
b. Gout
c. Rickets
d. Slipped disc

96. A type of diagnostic test used for cystitis is

a. ACTH
b. TSH
c. C & S
d. FBS

97. An individual with which type of blood can be a blood donor to individuals with any of the four blood types?

a. Type A
b. Type B
c. Type AB
d. Type O

98. An individual with which type of blood can receive all 4 blood types?

a. Type A
b. Type B
c. Type AB
d. Type O

99. The Rh factor is also known as the

a. A antigen
b. B antigen
c. AB antigen
d. D antigen

100. A condition marked by a decrease in the number of red blood cells is known as

a. Anemia
b. Leukemia
c. Thrombocytopenia
d. Polycythemia

101. The butterfly infusion set is used for all of the following types of patients EXCEPT

a. Infants
b. Obese patients
c. Adults with small wrists
d. Elderly patients

102. Which of the following statements regarding arterial puncture is FALSE?

a. The patient should be checked for allergies before the procedure
b. A patient afraid of needles should be calmed down
c. A phlebotomist may be trained to perform the procedure
d. The chance of a hematoma is increased

103. Intraoperative blood collection may be used in which type of surgery?

a. Transplant
b. Cancer
c. Lower GI tract
d. Pediatric

104. Which of the following statements regarding special blood collection procedures is FALSE?

a. Blood pressure cannot be performed on an AV shunt
b. Coagulation studies cannot be drawn from a heparin lock
c. A heparin lock may be left in the vein for 48 hours
d. An implanted port should be covered with a bandage

105. The proper pH level for arterial blood is

a. 5.35-5.45
b. 7.35-7.45
c. 3.35-3.45
d. 2.35-2.45

106. A patient's blood glucose level is usually elevated

a. After fasting
b. After ingesting a low-carbohydrate meal
c. After ingesting a high-carbohydrate meal
d. Two hours after ingesting a high-carbohydrate meal

107. The normal range for blood glucose level in a healthy adult is

a. 65-110 mg/dL
b. 45-65 mg/dL
c. 55-75 mg/dL
d. 45-90 mg/dL

108. The most plentiful electrolyte in serum or plasma is

a. Potassium
b. Sodium
c. Chloride
d. Calcium

109. Both sodium and potassium play a major role in

a. Osmotic pressure
b. Muscle function
c. Cardiac output
d. Renal function

110. Which of the following statements regarding HCG testing is FALSE?

a. Contaminants such as detergent may invalidate results
b. Medications may produce false-negative results
c. Positive results are available the first week after conception
d. Ovarian tumors may increase levels

111. Which of the following characteristics of a urine sample is indicative of a pathological condition?

a. White or pigmented yellow foam
b. Dark amber color
c. Epithelial cells
d. Bacteria

112. All of the following are indicative of a UTI EXCEPT

a. Leukocytes
b. Nitrites
c. Protein
d. Glucose

113. Trough levels are collected

a. 30 to 60 minutes after the drug is administered
b. To screen for drug intoxication
c. Prior to administration of the next dose
d. For DNA testing

114. TB is diagnosed using the

a. Schick test
b. PPD test
c. Dick test
d. Histo test

115. All of the following cannot be ingested prior to a fecal occult blood test EXCEPT

a. Vitamin C
b. Aspirin
c. Spinach
d. Horseradish

116. Which of the following is NOT normally present in the urine?

a. Ketones
b. Bilirubin
c. Albumin
d. Bacteria

117. Which of the following specimens must be kept at or near body temperature?

a. Lactic acid
b. Ammonia
c. Glucagon
d. Cryoglobulin

118. The ___ plane divides the body into top and bottom halves.

a. Sagittal
b. Midsagittal
c. Transverse
d. Frontal

119. The abbreviation Q2H indicates that the drug should be given

a. Twice a day
b. Every hour
c. By mouth
d. Every 2 hours

120. The most common type of tissue found in the body is

a. Connective
b. Muscle
c. Epithelial
d. Nerve

121. The total number of bones in the body is

a. 200
b. 100
c. 206
d. 106

122. The total number of muscles in the body is

a. 566
b. 656
c. 556
d. 560

123. The area between neurons over which impulses jump is known as the

a. Axon
b. Dendrite
c. Synapse
d. Myelin sheath

124. The gray matter of the brain is composed of

a. Myelin sheath
b. Nonmyelinated axons
c. Schwann cells
d. Synapses

125. The PNS is composed of

a. Cranial nerves
b. Optic nerves
c. Spinal cord
d. CNS

126. Hydrocephalus is characterized by

a. Stiff neck
b. Nerve pain
c. Shuffling gait
d. Enlarged head

127. The outermost layer of the skin is known as the

a. Dermis
b. Epidermis
c. Subcutaneous layer
d. Hypodermal layer

128. A condition characterized by protrusion of the stomach is known as

a. Gastritis
b. GERD
c. Hiatal hernia
d. Peptic ulcer

129. The __is a type of exocrine gland.

a. Pancreas
b. Pituitary
c. Thyroid
d. Sweat gland

130. Which of the following conditions is caused by dysfunction of the pituitary gland?

a. Cushing syndrome
b. Dwarfism
c. Diabetes
d. Parkinson disease

131. The throat is also known as the

a. Trachea
b. Larynx
c. Pharynx
d. Epiglottis

132. Asthma is caused by

a. Obstruction of the airway
b. Inflammation of the bronchial tubes
c. Too rapid breathing
d. Oxygen deficiency

133. The major portion of the heart is known as

a. Endocardium
b. Pericardium
c. Myocardium
d. Atrium

134. The pumping chambers of the heart are known as the

a. Ventricles
b. Atria
c. Endocardium
d. Septum

135. The human body has an average of _ pints of blood.

a. 4-5
b. 10-12
c. 8-10
d. 6-8

136. Approximately 92% of plasma is composed of

a. Fibrinogen
b. Solutes
c. Electrolytes
d. Water

137. A typical diagnostic test for cardiovascular disease is

a. CBC
b. Hgb
c. AST
d. ESR

138. The site typically used for testing ABGs is the

a. Venous puncture
b. Arterial puncture
c. Antecubital vein
d. Median cubital vein

139. Which type of urine specimen collection method is used in small children?

a. Clean catch
b. Midstream clean catch
c. Suprapubic
d. Regular void

140. All of the following may be used to test the CSF EXCEPT

a. Chloride
b. Total protein
c. Glucose
d. ABO

141. This specimen is collected 2 hours after the patient has ingested a meal

a. FBS
b. PP
c. Hgb
d. HBV

142. Which of the following tests may be performed together to assess clotting abnormalities?

a. ACT and PT
b. ACT and APPT
c. PT and PTT
d. PT and PP

143. Which of the following statements regarding the APPT test is FALSE?

a. Plasma values of 24 to 34 seconds are considered normal
b. Whole blood values are the same as plasma values
c. Whole blood values between 93 and 127 seconds are considered normal
d. Plasma values differ from whole blood values

144. Which of the following tests is typically ordered stat?

a. pCO2
b. HCG
c. FBS
d. Hgb

145. Enteric isolation procedures are required for

a. Patients with tuberculosis
b. Burn patients
c. Patients with intestinal infections
d. Patients with skin infections

146. OSHA requires that a HEPA respirator be used for

a. Enteric isolation
b. Burn patients
c. Contact isolation
d. AFB patients

147. SDS is required by OSHA for

a. Bloodborne pathogens
b. Electrical hazards
c. Hazardous chemicals
d. Radioactive hazards

148. Which of the following is NOT part of standard safety procedure?

a. Recapping contaminated needles
b. Replacing bed rails after specimen collection
c. Reporting items dropped on the floor
d. Reporting unusual odors

149. All of the following are required for pathogen growth EXCEPT

a. Water
b. Proper pH
c. Heat
d. Darkness

150. Postexposure treatment is recommended for

a. HCV
b. HBV
c. HIV
d. HBIG

151. Which of the following statements regarding HIV is FALSE?

a. HIV may be transmitted through breast milk
b. No vaccine is available for HIV
c. Postexposure treatment is recommended for occupational exposures
d. Those exposed to HIV must be retested 6 months after exposure

152. The source of transmission of a pathogen to others is known as the

a. Susceptible host
b. Reservoir host
c. Direct contact
d. Chain of infection

153. PPE is NOT required when entering the room of a patient with

a. Skin infection
b. Tuberculosis
c. Intestinal infection
d. HIV

154. Which of the following statements regarding laboratory hazards is FALSE?

a. Lead aprons should be worn as a precaution for radioactive hazards
b. Mixing bleach and ammonia creates a chemical hazard
c. All chemical exposures require flushing the eyes or affected parts with water
d. Electrical hazards should be removed using a broom handle

155. Which of the following information is NOT required on specimen tube labels?

a. Accession number
b. Physician's signature
c. Phlebotomist's initials
d. Time of test

156. All of the following are used to send laboratory requisition forms to the lab EXCEPT

a. Courier
b. Pneumatic tubes
c. E-mail
d. Verbal laboratory request

157. Which of the following statements regarding health care communication is FALSE?

a. Comfort zones are dependent on culture
b. Callers should not be put on hold
c. Sign language may be used for hearing-impaired patients
d. Sign language may be used for non–English-speaking patients

158. Which of the following constitutes negligence?

a. Intent to harm
b. Invasion of privacy
c. Injury
d. Abandonment

159. An example of an intentional tort is

a. Abandonment
b. Negligence
c. Malpractice
d. Chain of custody

160. Pre- and post- are examples of

a. Abbreviations
b. Suffixes
c. Prefixes
d. Root words

161. The term caudal means

a. Toward the midline
b. Toward the side
c. Toward the head
d. Toward the tail

162. Which of the following is NOT required for drug or alcohol testing?

a. Patient consent
b. Split sample
c. Plastic tube
d. Proctor

163. The ACT test is used to monitor

a. PO2
b. Heparin
c. Ionized calcium
d. Glucose

164. All of the following are trace elements EXCEPT

a. Arsenic
b. Zinc
c. Iron
d. Magnesium

165. Troponin is used in the diagnosis of

a. Diabetes
b. Heart attack
c. Anemia
d. Colon cancer

166. All of the following are skin tests EXCEPT

a. PPD
b. Histo
c. BNP
d. Cocci

167. In administering a TB test,

a. The antigen must be injected into a vein
b. The antigen must be injected just below the skin
c. The degree of erythema is measured to determine a reaction
d. Presence of a bleb or wheal indicates the antigen was injected improperly

168. A positive reaction to a TB test is indicated by

a. Induration between 5 and 9 mm in diameter
b. Induration less than 5 mm in diameter
c. Induration greater than 10 mm in diameter
d. Degree of erythema

169. All of the following are included in the procedure for strep testing EXCEPT

a. Latex agglutination
b. Nitrous acid extraction
c. Enzyme immunoassay
d. Specific gravity

170. Which of the following statements regarding arterial puncture is FALSE?

a. Arterial puncture is more difficult to perform than venipuncture
b. Arterial puncture is used to evaluate ABGs
c. Arterial puncture is used for routine blood tests
d. Arterial puncture is more painful than venipuncture

171. Decreased levels in the blood, as measured by one of the following, increase the respiration rate.

a. PCO2
b. PO2
c. HCO3
d. pH

172. Base excess or deficit is calculated based on all of the following EXCEPT

a. PCO2
b. HCO3
c. Hct
d. O2 saturation

173. Which of the following statements regarding the radial artery is FALSE?

a. The radial artery may be difficult to locate in patients with low cardiac output
b. If the radial artery is damaged, the ulnar artery may be used for arterial puncture
c. The radial artery should not be punctured in the absence of collateral circulation
d. The radial artery carries a higher risk of hematoma

174. The femoral artery is located in the

a. Groin
b. Scalp
c. Arm
d. Umbilical cord

175. In performing the Allen test,

a. The patient should hyperextend the fingers
b. Blanching of the hand indicates a positive result
c. Both the radial and ulnar arteries should be compressed at the same time
d. Only the radial artery should be compressed

176. In infants, which of the following sites may be used for arterial puncture?

a. Brachial artery
b. Umbilical artery
c. Femoral artery
d. Ulnar artery

177. The presence of a wheal indicates

a. Proper injection of a local anesthetic
b. Positive TB test
c. Positive Allen test
d. Improper injection of the TB antigen

178. The vasovagal response is commonly known as

a. Allergic reaction
b. Myocardial infarction
c. Fainting
d. Hematoma

179. Serous fluid may be obtained from all of the following EXCEPT the

a. Peritoneal cavity
b. Pleural cavity
c. Pericardial cavity
d. Spinal cavity

180. The C-urea breath test is used to detect

a. Lactose intolerance
b. H pylori
c. Trace metals
d. Blood disorders

Answer Key and Explanations

1. D: All of the above. Receiving cannot accession a specimen without:

- A label that clearly states the patient's name, collection date, doctor's name and contact information, specimen type, and test required.
- An uncontaminated, valid requisition bearing the doctor's signature, patient's billing information, and pertinent information (acute or convalescent phase, antibiotic use, fever, or traveler).
- Intact specimen container.
- Correct media type or preservative used for the specimen type.
- Same-day collection date, or preincubated at room temperature or subcultivated, and then vented, to prevent false-negatives of nonfermentative species.
- If the specimen does not meet these conditions, call the doctor's office and get the missing information. Discard the specimen if you cannot obtain full information, and inform the doctor's office that recollection is required.

2. A: 120 gallons of class I, II, and IIIA liquids. Choice A complies with fire safety standards. Class IA, IB, and IC are flammables. Class II, IIIA, and IIIB are combustibles. No more than 120 gallons of class I, II, and IIIA liquids can be stored in a lab fridge, and of those, no more than 60 gallons may be class I and II. Do not locate more than three storage cabinets in one fire area. No more than 50% of the flammables can be stored for teaching. Use DOT-approved glass, metal, or polyethylene containers no larger than 1.1 gallons (4 L).

3. A: How probable it is a patient will develop a disease, and its etiology. A is correct because disease incidence measures how prevalent a disease is among a given population in a specific place, over a specific time. Incidence predicts how probable it is a patient will develop a disease, and its etiology (likely cause). Choices B, C, and D are incorrect because they refer to a related concept called predicted values, which estimate how likely a test result is to be right or wrong, given certain variables, such as the patient's age, occupation, race, income, how long the symptoms have lasted, and if there is fever.

4. B: Only applies if absorbance is between 0.1 and 1.0. B is correct because Beer's law states absorbance is proportional to the concentration of a solution, but Beer's law only applies if absorbance is between 0.1 and 1.0. Different substances absorb different light wavelengths, so a spectrophotometer (Spec-20) compares the intensity of light entering a sample and exiting from it (percent transmittance) to find the concentration of the sample. A completely transparent sample has 100% transmittance. A completely opaque sample has 0% transmittance. Visible spectrum light ranges from 440 nm to 700 nm.

5. C: Presumptive identification. C is correct. Note the color, outline (circular, rhizoid, or wavy), elevation (convex, flat, or raised), and translucency (opaque, translucent, or transparent) for presumptive identification. Differential identification means naming bacteria according to their headspace gases and volatile compounds they release as they grow on media, with a spectrometer (microDMx). Adanson's numerical taxonomy (phonetics) ranks microorganisms according to how similar they are genetically and morphologically. Closely related bacteria form a cluster, which is classified into objective, repeatable taxa. TaqMan, SWOrRD, and MicroSeq are quick screening kits. They are not as accurate as cultures but are quicker when time is critical. Polymerase chain reaction (PCR) in quick kits amplifies the genetic material, and then the 1450 base pair region of the 16S rDNA gene is sequenced by electrophoresis.

6. B: Toxicology. Serology/Immunology studies antibodies in the liquid part of blood. Cytology studies cells for cancer, such as Pap smears. Endocrinology studies hormones, such as diabetes and acromegaly.

7. C: Normal hemoglobin. Hemoglobin electrophoresis differentiates hemoglobin into normal HbA and normal HbA2, or abnormal HbS in sickle cell patients, or HbC in hemolytic anemia patients, or HbF in a fetus or newborn.

8. A: Sensitivity. Sensitivity (recall rate) measures how many times a test produces true-positive results, which indicates patients probably have a disease, compared with the gold standard test for that particular illness. Sensitivity allows early detection of disease and prevents epidemics. Divide the number of patients who definitely have the disease and test positive by the total patients tested who have the disease (including those who tested false-negative), and multiply by 100 to obtain the percentage sensitivity. Specificity measures how many times a test produces true-negative results, meaning patients probably do not have a disease, compared with the gold standard test for that particular illness. Specificity is important for cancer chemotherapy and other toxic treatments. Aliquot is dividing a solution into equal parts. Aliquot allows very expensive reagents or drugs, and blood samples that are below scale, to be used efficiently. Circadian rhythm is a normal daily flow that affects hormones, which are normally higher in the morning than in the afternoon.

9. C: Green, gray, and marbled SST blood collection tubes Hematology requires mostly lavender, light blue, and black tubes. Blood Bank and Public Health require red, pink, and yellow tubes. Toxicology requires navy, purple, and brown tubes. If you draw the wrong color tube, it contains an inappropriate anticoagulant, and the test will be invalidated.

10. A: BUN to Creatinine ratio between 15:1 and 20:1. Blood urea nitrogen (BUN) and creatinine are waste products of protein metabolism, measured in kidney function tests performed with a 24-hour urine. If the kidneys do not filter properly, creatinine output in the urine decreases, and creatine blood levels increase. High creatinine (more than 1.5 mg/dL) and BUN (more than 20 mg/dL) means the patient has a kidney disease (e.g., glomerulonephritis, pyelonephritis, stones, tubular necrosis, tumors). BUN and creatinine must be in correct proportion for optimal health. ALP and AST are liver function tests. Amylase is a pancreas test.

11. D: All of the above. Newborn jaundice is different from adult jaundice. Babies have more red blood cells and reticulocytes than adults do. Babies have immature livers that are not yet efficient at breaking down bilirubin. Adult jaundice is usually from hepatitis or cirrhosis of the liver. Erythroblastosis fetalis means the baby's Rh factor is incompatible with his mother's Rh, leading to hemolytic disease of the newborn. Kernicterus means the bilirubin is greater than 5 mg/dL, resulting in hemolytic anemia if not treated with phototherapy (blue lights). Physiologic jaundice occurs in breastfed babies released from the hospital too early and without a vitamin K injection, but resolves in a week with adequate fluids.

12. B: Triglycerides. Anions are negatively charged ions of chloride and bicarbonate. Cholesterol is lipids from animal sources that climb after a fatty meal. An eluent is a solvent used for chromatography.

13. C: Protein electrophoresis. The serum proteins test includes total protein, albumin, and globulin. Ascites is swelling of the abdomen from extra fluid in the peritoneum, resulting from end-stage diseases of the heart, kidney, liver, ovary, and pancreas. When serum proteins make the doctor suspect one of these diseases, the doctor follows up with protein electrophoresis. Four globulin fractionations are added to the total protein and albumin: alpha-1 globulin, alpha-2 globulin, beta globulin, and gamma globulin. Electrophoresis patterns and the patient's history of drug use help pinpoint the diagnosis, which may extend to rheumatoid arthritis, muscle tumors, and immune deficiencies. Bilirubin is the brownish-red bile pigment from broken down blood cells in the liver.

14. A: Alcoholism, hypothyroidism, cardioversion, or clofibrate use. Cardiac enzymes elevate soon after a heart attack, but that is not the only possible root cause. CPK elevates in alcoholism; cardiac catheterization; stroke; clofibrate use; electric shock applied during resuscitation; low thyroid hormone and high thyroid-stimulating hormone; and after surgery. B and D refer to situations that cause AST enzyme to rise. C refers to situations that cause LDH enzyme to rise.

15. D: Cushing syndrome. Cortisol is an adrenal stress hormone that is normally higher around 8:00 in the morning (6 to 28 mcg/dL) and lower at 4:00 in the afternoon (2 to 12 mcg/dL). The fluctuation is a normal diurnal variation. Cushing syndrome patients have sustained high cortisol. Addison's disease patients have chronically low cortisol levels, diagnosed by a 24-hour urine test for 17-hydroxycorticosteroids. Abnormal cortisol levels also appear in thyroid and pituitary gland disease, obesity, and cancer, and when steroids, diuretics, or birth control pills are used, but it is not the same pattern as Cushing syndrome. B refers to atrial natriuretic factor (ANF), produced by the heart's atria during volume overload and high blood pressure.

16. B: Hyponatremia, often from vomiting and diarrhea, furosemide, or Addison's disease. Hyponatremia results from too much water and not enough salt in the bloodstream. Hyponatremia often presents as a urine sample with a specific gravity (SG) lower than the normal 1.015 to 1.025 and closer to the SG of water (1.000). Hypernatremia refers to too much salt in the bloodstream, which increases SG above 1.025. Hyperkalemia and hypokalemia refer to the level of potassium, not sodium.

17. A: Rise 6 hours after heart attack, peak in 18 hours, and return to baseline in 3 days. CPK is the first enzyme to rise following a heart attack, so doctors measure it before the other cardiac enzymes. If creatine kinase-MB (CK-MB) rises, it means the heart sustained severe damage. B. refers to the response of AST to a heart attack. C refers to the response of LDH to a heart attack. D does not apply because alpha-fetoprotein (AFP) is used to find liver disease, testicular cancer, and birth defects.

18. A: 120 days. A normal erythrocyte (red blood cell [RBC]) lives for four months. When it wears out, the spleen destroys it and the liver converts it to bilirubin, which the gallbladder stores as bile and the digestive system uses to break down dietary fats. Old red blood cells puff into a sphere, rather than retaining their original barbell-shape. Changing shape makes them fragile and inflexible. Babies have 4.8 to 7.2 million RBCs per cubic millimeter of blood. Adult males have 4 to 6 million, and adult females 4 to 5 million RBCs. Pregnant women have lower RBC counts.

19. D: Rouleaux formation. Normal red blood cells settle slowly when standing in a test tube: males 0 to 15 millimeters per hour; females 0 to 20 mm/h; children 0 to 10 mm/h; elderly patients 5 to 10 mm/h more. A low sedimentation rate indicates hemorrhage. A high sedimentation rate indicates cells are heavier and falling quicker than normal, usually from inflammatory diseases, parasite infection, cell death, heavy metal poisoning, or toxemia of pregnancy. However, cold agglutinins also make red blood cells adhere to each other in a Rouleaux formation when they are chilled.

20. C: Leukocyte alkaline phosphatase (LAP). Hematologists use LAP stain to highlight neutrophils when the patient has many white blood cells but not leukemia (leukemic reaction). Microbiologists use periodic acid-Schiff (PAS) to stain carbohydrates, collagen, fibrin, and mucin purple. Sudan black B (SBB) is specifically for acute leukemia patients; it helps to differentiate between immature cells by staining lipids in myeloid leukemia that are absent in lymphoid leukemia. LPCB is mixed with 10% potassium hydroxide (KOH) to identify fungus.

21. D: Both a and c.Make a bone marrow slide with a battlement technique so the review is more standardized, with even cell distribution. Wedge push technique (feathered end) causes the white cells to pool unevenly on the slide. On the side edges and in the feather of a wedge push slide, you will find concentrated pockets of eosinophils, monocytes, and segmented neutrophils. Small lymphocytes concentrate in the center of the slide.

22. A: Phase I problems. Phase I of coagulation happens in the first 3 to 5 minutes after an injury, when the platelets mobilize. Factor III distress call is sent in phase II, not phase I. Factor VIII deficiency is the problem that causes hemophilia. Fibrinolysis occurs when the injured site is plugged with a blood clot and plasminogen changes to plasmin.

23. B: Lupus inhibitor antibody (LA). Hematologists use phospholipid in PT and PTT tests to check how fast a patient clots. The normal range for PTT is 60 to 70 seconds. Lupus inhibitor antibody (LA) acts against the phospholipid and falsely extends clotting time. LA is implicated in miscarriages, rheumatoid arthritis, lupus, Reynaud syndrome, and thromboembolism. Platelet antibody testing is only appropriate if the patient has purpura and hemoglobinuria. Intrinsic factor is incorrect; it is the stomach's ability to produce B12 to prevent pernicious anemia.

24. B: Fungal serology titer of more than 1:32 that increases x4 or more 3 weeks later. First, gently scrape suspected fungus off the patient's skin. Mix two drops of 10% potassium hydroxide (KOH) and one drop of LPCB on a glass slide, cover it, and warm it to observe budding yeasts. Add a drop of calcofluor white before warming to see fluorescent infected tissue. Put a drop of India ink on a wet mount to see clear cryptococcal capsules. Confirm the microscopic exam with fungal serology when you test the skin scraping and again in three weeks. The doctor may follow up by ordering latex serology for cryptococcal antigen to find meningitis, complement fixation for coccidiomycosis and histoplasmosis, and immunodiffusion for blastomycosis.

25. A: Plasmacrit test (PCT) and rapid plasma reagin (RPR) test. The old screening test for syphilis is VDRL, which measures Treponema pallidum antibodies by flocculation reaction to the diphosphatidyl glycerol in ox heart extract. However, VDRL misses cases of syphilis that are less than four weeks old, and half of cases that are in the late stages. VDRL is not very sensitive, and often gives a false-positive result for patients with the following conditions: pregnancy, hepatitis, HIV, leprosy, lupus (SLE), Lyme disease, malaria, mononucleosis, pneumonia, rheumatic fever, or rheumatoid arthritis. PCT and RCR are less likely to be confounded, and since they require less blood, are replacing VDRL. ELISA confirms syphilis infection by identifying the specific antibodies. FTA-ABS is 100% accurate for secondary syphilis, but it is expensive, and the patient will always test positive once infected. Captia is required to confirm RPR. Cold agglutinins increase in children with congenital syphilis.

26. D: Dilute 1 mL of serum with 1 mL of saline. You must know how to dilute to perform a titer, which measures how many times a blood sample must be diluted with saline before an antibody can no longer be found in it. First, check the antibody/antigen reaction against the controls with undiluted serum. To prevent blood clotting (Rouleaux formation) during dilution, warm the blood and saline to body temperature (37°C) for 10 minutes before diluting. Dilute 1 mL of serum with 1 mL of saline for a dilution of ½, or 1:2. Pipette off 1 mL of this dilution into an aliquot tube. Add 1 mL of saline, and it becomes a 1:4 dilution. If you dilute up to 1:32 and get no reaction, the end-point titer is 16.

27. A: Guinea pig, cow, and horse. Monospot heterophile antibodies test confirms an early infection of mononucleosis, caused by Epstein-Barr virus. If the infection is older than 9 weeks, then the doctor orders EBV antibody test. On a glass slide, mix a drop of the patient's blood with guinea pig kidney antigen to absorb Forssman antibodies. Add beef red blood stroma to absorb non-Forssman antibodies. Mix with horse blood. Guinea pig agglutination means the patient has early mononucleosis. Beef should not agglutinate. Monospot can be false-negative on children younger than 10, or before two weeks of infection. B, C, and D are not applicable to Monospot.

28. C: Both syphilis and HIV. Patients coinfected with HIV and syphilis are immunosuppressed. When performing a titer to find antibodies in an HIV/syphilitic, beware prozone phenomenon. The coinfected patient's undiluted serum may produce a false-negative result because it does not agglutinate. Alternatively, it may show very little agglutination at low dilutions, but agglutinates more at higher dilutions because of excess antibodies. Monospot is used to find EBV mononucleosis. Reynaud disease is characterized by rouleaux formation and high cold agglutinin titers. IgG occurs in patients who are convalescing from mononucleosis.

29. D: Both a and b.. RhoGAM is the brand name for Rh immunoglobulin. It is administered to Rh- women who acquired anti-D antibodies from a previous blood transfusion or pregnancy. The infant and father do not receive RhoGAM at all. If there is a live birth, the mother gets 300 mcg of RhoGAM during week 26 to 28 of her pregnancy, and again before her infant is 3 days old. If the pregnancy miscarries before week 13 or is aborted, then the mother gets a lower dose of 50 mcg of MICRhoGAM. If the miscarriage or abortion happens after week 13, use RhoGAM.

30. A: Eosinophilia, hypocalcemia, leukopenia, and pancytopenia may occur. The first lab sign of a mild transfusion reaction is the oxyhemoglobin dissociation curve shifts left. Later, the number of eosinophils will increase and the calcium level will drop. Finally, white blood cells will decrease, and then all blood cells will decrease. Minimize the chance of transfusion reaction by washing the donor's red blood cells in sterile normal saline before transfusion. If the doctor anticipates a mild transfusion reaction, he/she may give antihistamines to the patient before transfusion, and may order the removal of white cells from the bag of blood by a Sepacell R-500 leukocyte reduction filter. Irradiated blood products prevent fatal transfusion-associated graft-versus-host disease (TA-GVHD). The safest way for a patient to prepare for elective surgery is to bank his own blood for transfusion (autologous donation).

31. C: No A or B antigens and both anti-A and anti-B antibodies. Type O- blood is the universal donor because it has no A or B antigens, or Rh+ antibodies. If there is no time to crossmatch a trauma patient, then O– blood is given without compatibility testing to prevent death. A routine type and cross takes 45 minutes and the delay could be fatal.

32. B: Trauma patient with hemoglobin of 5 g/dL. Blood Bank triages patients in the following priority sequence: (1) emergency trauma victims with isovolemic anemia from hemorrhage; (2) surgical patients who lose more than 3 cups of blood; (3) regular users of coagulation factors. If you anticipate a blood shortage because of a massive trauma, then contact the nurse manager as soon as possible. The surgical team may decide to cancel elective surgery, or delay it until the patient is medically treated to reduce anemia. If surgery must proceed, the surgical team may consider the following blood conservation methods if you warn them ahead of time: erythropoietin, autologous donations, or hemodilution before surgery; cell savers, hypotension, electrocautery, and lasers during surgery; and administering antifibrinolytics after surgery.

33. D: All of the above. A type and cross is very time-consuming (45 minutes) and must meet very specific safety standards to avoid a transfusion reaction. All of the following conditions must be met:

- Specimens labeled at the patient's bedside with full name or the emergency department identification number; initials are unacceptable. Specimens must not have pink serum. Donor blood must not be clotted, fatty, or contaminated.
- Patient wears an identification band, which is checked at collection and transfusion times. The band must not be taped to the bed. The patient's name and a unique identification number (Blood Bank identification number, hospital number, health insurance number, or unique lifetime identifier) must appear on the band, in case there is a patient with a similar name.
- Requisitions must bear the collector's and identifier's names, collection date and time (in case antibodies develop), the ordering doctor's name, the amount and type of blood requested, the patient's date of birth (if known), relevant patient history (e.g., pregnant and bleeding; signs of transfusion reaction).

34. A: Midstream urine collection (MSU). MSU is required to diagnose cystitis and pyelitis accurately. Witnessed collection is only required for drug testing. 24-hour urines are for hormone tests. Random urine may have contamination, so while it is suitable for chemistry, random urine is inaccurate for microbiology. Collect midstream urine any time of day, in a sterile, lidded container. Your microbiologist may want the patient to use a benzalkonium chloride wipe before collection. Without a wipe, the sample is not a clean catch. Do not touch the inside of the container, as it contaminates the specimen and produces a false-positive.

35. A: Cell count, glucose and protein, gram stain and culture, virology/mycology/cytology. Only a physician can collect cerebrospinal fluid (CSF) from a lumbar puncture. The MLT just prepares a collection tray and assists as ordered. The tray must contain the following: iodine prep; alcohol prep; 3 cc of 1% lidocaine; 25g, 5/8" needle; 22g, 1.5" needle; atraumatic spinal needle (to prevent postcollection headache); syringe; four sterile red stoppered tubes; 4x4 gauze; sponge forceps; sterile towels; small basin; and a Band-Aid. The physician collects the fluid between L3 and L4 in the patient's spine and hands you the tubes. Label one tube each for cell count, glucose and protein, gram stain and culture, and virology/mycology/cytology. You only need a fifth tube if the physician wants globulin immunoelectrophoresis, which is rare. C and D tests are included in A, and it is unnecessary to requisition them separately.

36. C: Pyorrhea and Lemierre syndrome. The pathogenic phyla are xenobacteria, cyanobacteria, firmicutes, flavobacteria, fusobacteria, planctomycetes, proteobacteria, spirochaetes, and verrucomicrobia. Planctomycetes causes chlamydia and pneumonia. Spirochaetes cause Lyme disease. Proteobacteria causes stomach ulcers. Firmicutes cause food poisoning. Fusobacteria cause pockets of pus in the gums that can break off into septic blood clots in the jugular vein of the neck. The septic clots can travel to cause abscesses in distant parts of the body, such as the brain, joints, kidney, and liver. Lemierre syndrome from gum disease was common until the discovery of antibiotics.

37. D: Löwenstein-Jensen (LJ) egg. TB is a fussy bacterium to grow in the lab and requires egg media. Tinsdale is used to find C. diphtheria. Sheep blood is used to find slow-growing anaerobic bacteria. MYW is used to find Legionella pneumonia. It is important for the MLT to know what type of infection the doctor suspects, so the correct media can be used for culture. Failure to pick the correct media may result in a false-negative and the disease will go undiagnosed.

38. B: 10x. To find parasites such as worms, set the microscope's magnification to 10x. Parasites often cause bleeding, so set the microscope to 40x to find the blood cells. Higher powers are unnecessary to view animal parasites and count cells, and would just slow down the MLT's reading of the slide. Calibrate the ocular micrometer every time a new technician is hired, each time you change optics, and annually thereafter.

39. A: Crypto (Cryptosporidium parvum). In the United States, the lab technician is required by law to report the following nine parasites to Public Health authorities if they are found in patient samples: Cryptosporidium parvum, Cyclospora cayetanensis, Entamoeba histolytica, hematoxylin, Giardia duodenalis, Plasmodium falciparum, Taenia, Trichinella spiralis, and Enterobius vermicularis. Hookworm, tapeworm, and pinworm are very common infestations and do not need to be reported. Your lab must provide reference slides or a parasite atlas for you to compare against the patients' specimens. Keep positive specimens in your lab for at least one year, either as a permanently stained slide, or as a preserved stool sample that is safely stored. Public Health may order them for examination.

40. D: Wet mount fresh, liquid stool with LPCB stain. Giardia lamblia is a parasite that lives in the small intestine of humans who consume contaminated food or water. Giardia causes traveler's diarrhea. Giardia cysts are activated by stomach acid and become trophozoites. The MLT can get the patient to swallow a string for several hours and then examine it for trophozoites, but many patients are uncooperative and prefer to leave a stool sample instead. To prepare the wet mount, strain well-formed stool. Concentrate it in the centrifuge at 2000 rpm for 4 minutes in a conical tube. Ream the tube with a wooden stick. Add 10% formalin. Make a tan suspension. You should be able to read a newspaper through the slide. Examine microscopically at 10x for parasites and 40x for blood. Use an ocular micrometer to measure parasites. Mix stool with PVA plastic powder to glue it onto the slide before permanent staining with iodine or Snap n' Stain.

41. B: One year. Parasites are a serious Public Health issue. It is important to prevent parasites acquired in foreign countries from spreading through the American populace. Even though you check your patient's specimen against reference slides or a parasite atlas, you could miss rare species or misidentify the parasite in its different stages of development. A Public Health official has the right to check your slide for one year after initial testing. To ensure your test is accurate, use positive and negative controls to check your antigens every time you receive a new shipment and every month thereafter. Use the right stain for the right specimen. Refrigerate stool within three hours of receiving it, if you do not have time to fix it with preservative.

42. D: Mycology specimens. The MLT uses a Wood's lamp to help identify fungus on the patient's skin before collecting it. Fungus will fluoresce bright lime green under the Wood's light, so the MLT will find it easily and can scrape it off with a tongue depressor into a sterile container for testing. Malaria parasites are found in blood smears. Public Health specimens are usually blood serology or stool for parasites. Toxicology specimens are usually red, navy, or purple stoppered blood tubes for drugs or heavy metals.

43. D: Nitrites. There is a nitrite pad on an N-Multistix for routine urinalysis. Some bacteria eat nitrates in urine, and shed nitrites as a waste product. E. coli is one of the bacteria detectable by nitrites in urine. However, not finding nitrites does not mean there is no infection. For example, strep is a very serious and common kidney infection, but does not produce nitrites. Leukocytes indicate an infection in a person with a healthy immune system, but an immunosuppressed patient may not produce leukocytes in urine. Protein indicates kidney damage, but it is not necessarily from an infection. Ketones are a byproduct of fat metabolism that appear in diabetic patients and crash dieters.

44. A: Testicular cancer. Do not assume that the doctor filled out the wrong name and sex on the requisition if you receive a request for a pregnancy test on a man. A pregnancy test looks for the hormone beta-human chorionic gonadotropin (hCG). A pregnant woman excretes beta-hCG 10 days after conceiving a child. However, a male with carcinoma of the testicles also excretes this same pregnancy hormone. Normal males never excrete beta-hCG. If your patient had an orchiectomy (removal of the testicles) but is still excreting beta-hCG in a follow-up test, then metastasized cancer is present. The doctor must remove it surgically, or with radiation or chemotherapy. Prostatitis would produce leukocytes but not hCG. Cryptorchidism is undescended testicles, which can lead to cancer in later life. Peyronie disease is a bent penis from scar tissue, and does not produce hCG.

45. D: 750 to 2,000 mL. A patient should produce at least 500 mL (2 cups) of urine each and every day. Ideally, a patient should produce 750 mL (3 cups) to 2,000 mL (5 cups) of urine to maintain good health. If the patient has vomiting and diarrhea, or an enlarged prostate gland or severe infection, or uses too much medication, then he will produce scanty urine (oliguria). Some of the drug overdoses that decrease urinary output are anticholinergics, methotrexate, and diuretics. Patients whose kidneys are failing have anuria, which strictly interpreted means absence of urine, but they actually produce 100 mL or less of urine per day. Patients who have diabetes insipidus or diabetes mellitus often produce far too much urine (3½ quarts or more). They are very thirsty and may drink more than a gallon of fluid per day (more than 12 glasses). The antidepressant lithium is one drug that can cause frequent urination as an adverse effect.

46. C: Gout. Patients with gout have extreme pain in their great toes due to needles of uric acid crystals that form around their joints. Patients with struvite crystals in their urine have bacterial infections. Patients with tyrosine or cystine crystals in their urine may be poisoned or have a serious metabolic disorder. Patients with phosphate or calcium oxalate crystals in their urine have too much parathyroid hormone or malabsorption. Crystals do not appear in healthy urine.

47. C: Hematuria and uroliths. Polycystic kidney disease is an inherited disorder that produces bloody urine and kidney stones. It is the most common inherited disease in the United States, and it is the fourth leading cause of kidney failure. Cysts may also appear in the patient's liver, but do not produce cirrhosis or hepatitis. Destruction of the kidney does eventually produce high blood pressure, but the PKD patient is a poor candidate for a bypass graft because of abnormal heart valves. The patient may develop abnormal pockets in the intestine that fill with hard stool (diverticulosis); however, they seldom produce severe bleeding. Melena is a tarry, black stool caused by internal bleeding, and hematochezia is red stools caused by heavy bleeding.

48. B: Droplet transmission involves transfer of an infectious agent via droplets larger than 5 μm in diameter, whereas airborne transmission involves dispersal of infectious evaporated droplet nuclei less than 5 μm in diameter. In vector transmission, infectious agents are carried by insects, arthropods, or animals; in vehicle transmission, infectious agents are transmitted through contaminated food, water, or drugs.

49. C: The transmission of bubonic plague by fleas from rodents is an example of vector transmission; tuberculosis is spread via airborne transmission. Transmission of salmonella infection associated with handling contaminated food and human immunodeficiency virus (HIV) infection through blood transfusion are examples of vehicle transmission.

50. D: Droplet transmission may result from transfer of infectious agents by coughing, sneezing, or talking or through procedures such as throat swab collection. Vector transmission may result from mosquito or flea bites and vehicle transmission though contaminated food or water; transfer of an infectious agent through kissing or touching is known as direct contact transmission.

51. A: Routine hand washing using plain soap and water is required to prevent spread of infection; alcohol-based antiseptic hand cleaners may also be used. Artificial nails or nails longer than one quarter inch are prohibited. After hand washing, a clean paper towel should be used to turn off the faucet to prevent contamination.

52. C: Protective or reverse isolation may be required for patients highly susceptible to infection, such as burn patients, patients with AIDS, or chemotherapy patients with a low neutrophil count; protective isolation is usually not required for infants.

53. A: Never use both hands to recap a needle; hands should be washed both before putting on and after removing gloves. Standard precautions should be followed for all body fluids except sweat; resuscitation devices may be used as an alternative to mouth-to-mouth resuscitation.

54. C: An N95 respirator must be worn by all individuals susceptible to measles or chickenpox before entering the room of a patient known or suspected to have these diseases; however, adults who are immune to measles or chickenpox are not required to wear an N95 respirator or surgical mask.

55. D: Shoulder-length or longer hair is acceptable in the laboratory if it is tied back; wearing nail polish or large or dangling earrings is not acceptable. A laboratory coat should never be worn when leaving the lab for any reason.

56. C: HBV vaccine does not contain live virus and thus does not carry the risk of HBV infection; HBV vaccine also protects against hepatitis D virus (HDV) because it is only contracted concurrently with HBV. HBV can survive up to 1 week in dried blood on work surfaces or other objects.

57. B: Hepatitis C virus (HCV) infection may occur through exposure to blood and serum and is primarily transmitted through sexual contact and needle sharing; however, it is rarely found in urine or semen and is not associated with phlebotomy procedures.

58. C: Cleansing the wound with plain soap and water for at least 30 seconds is useful in reducing the risk of transmission of a bloodborne pathogen; squeezing the wound or cleansing the wound with an antiseptic, bleach, or other caustic agents is not recommended.

59. B: A specific class of fire extinguisher is used for each class of fire except for class D fires; these types of fires involve combustible or reactive metals such as sodium, potassium, magnesium, or lithium and should be handled by trained firefighting personnel.

60. A: Class K fires are often caused by high-temperature cooking oils, grease, or fats; class A fires occur with wood, paper, or clothing and class B fires with flammable liquids and vapors such as paint or gasoline. Class D fires are associated with combustible or reactive materials such as sodium or potassium.

61. C: When adding additional compresses to a wound, the original compress should not be removed to avoid interference with the clotting process; direct pressure should be applied to the wound using cloth or gauze. An elastic bandage can be used to hold the compress in place.

62. B: IV is an acceptable acronym; however, IU, or international unit, is often confused with IV and thus should not be used. U should be written out as "unit" and QD as "daily."

63. B: A patient lying on their stomach is in the prone position; a patient lying on their back, face up, is in the supine position. A patient standing erect with arms at their sides and palms facing forward is considered to be in the anatomic position. Reclined position is also referred to as semi-Fowler's position, with the head of the bed at approximately 30 to 45 degrees.

64. C: Because the spinal cord ends at the first lumbar vertebra, lumbar puncture does not present a risk of spinal cord injury. The physician inserts the needle into the spinal cavity at the space between the 3rd and 4th lumbar vertebrae.

65. A: The hormone epinephrine increases heart rate, blood pressure, and metabolic rate; the antidiuretic hormone (ADH) decreases urine production and calcitonin lowers blood calcium levels. Melatonin helps set diurnal rhythms and is associated with seasonal affective disorder (SAD).

66. C: Increased levels of creatine kinase (CK) are associated with heart attack; PSA, or prostate specific antigen, level is used to test for prostate cancer. Carcinoembryonic antigen (CEA) is used in digestive system testing and albumin in urinary system testing.

67. A: In the recommended order of draw for syringes, sterile specimens are first, followed by light-blue tops; the SST follows the red top and the gray-top tube is last.

68. C: According to the alternate syringe order of draw, the sterile specimens remain first, while the red top and SST tubes are last.

69. D: A sign with a picture of falling leaves indicates that fall precautions are required for the patient. The letters DNR indicate a do not resuscitate order, and a sign depicting a delete symbol over an arm with a needlestick indicates no blood pressures in right arm.

70. C: Occasionally, the name of the ordering physician, room number, or bed number on the patient's ID band may differ; however, patient identity must always be verified before collecting blood. As part of informed consent, patients have the right to refuse blood draw; thus, the phlebotomist must ask the patient's permission before collecting blood.

71. C: The phlebotomist should always verify a patient's ID, even if he or she has been identified by the receptionist or has responded when his or her name has been called. Some outpatients may have been issued an ID card by the clinic; however, outpatients should still be asked to confirm their name and date of birth.

72. B: Because the median cubital vein is closer to the surface and located in an area least prone to nerve damage, it is the preferred site for venipuncture. The cephalic and median cephalic veins are the second choice; the basilic and median basilic veins are least preferred because of their proximity to the median nerve and brachial artery.

73. A: When applying a tourniquet, fist pumping should be discouraged, as it may make vein location more difficult or cause changes in blood components that may affect test results. A tourniquet may be applied over a patient's sleeve if the sleeve is too tight and cannot be rolled up far enough; a tourniquet should never be placed over an open sore. Because a tourniquet may have a tendency to roll or twist on the arm of an obese patient, two tourniquets may be placed on top of each other and used together.

74. B: If an antecubital vein cannot be found on either arm, a capillary puncture may be considered provided the test can be performed on capillary blood. Veins on the underside of the wrist should not be used to avoid nerve injury; tendons should not be used as they are difficult to penetrate and lack resilience. Manipulating the site may change blood composition, which may interfere with test results.

75. A: Because outpatient specimens are not obtained during the basal state, normal values may differ slightly from those of inpatients; hemoglobin (Hgb), hematocrit (Hct), and red blood cell (RBC) counts may have higher normal ranges at higher elevations. Caffeinated beverages may affect cortisol levels; ingestion of lipids such as butter or cheese may increase blood lipid content, giving blood specimens a cloudy or milky appearance.

76. D: Blood glucose levels are usually lowest in the morning; however, iron, insulin, and potassium levels are usually highest in the morning.

77. C: Exercise may increase levels of protein, insulin, glucose, and cholesterol, as well as skeletal muscle enzyme levels, but does not affect liver enzyme levels.

78. C: Body position, environmental conditions such as temperature and humidity, and stress can affect blood specimen composition; fasting is useful in eliminating dietary influences on blood testing.

79. A: Venipuncture should never be performed through a hematoma; if there is no alternative, an area distal to the hematoma should be used. In patients with a tattoo, it is best to choose another site; however, if there is no alternative, the needle should be inserted in an area that does not contain dye. In a mastectomy patient, blood should not be drawn from the arm on the same side of the mastectomy, but can be drawn from the other arm. Pregnancy does not preclude blood collection.

80. C: If a patient faints during blood collection, discontinue the draw and discard the needle; pressure should be applied to the site to prevent bleeding and bruising and the patient should be asked to lower his or her head and breathe deeply to allow oxygenated blood to access the brain. Ammonia inhalants may produce side effects such as respiratory distress in asthmatic patients and should not be used. After he or she regains consciousness, the patient should remain in the room for at least 15 minutes.

81. D: Petechiae, or small red spots that appear on the patient's skin when the tourniquet is applied, are usually caused by capillary wall defects or platelet abnormalities and are indicative of heavy bleeding at the venipuncture site; however, they are not indicative of hematoma. Using veins that are too small or fragile for the size of the needle, applying inadequate pressure to the site, and allowing the needle to penetrate all the way through the vein may cause hematoma formation.

82. B: To prevent hemoconcentration during venipuncture, the phlebotomist should ask the patient to release his or her fist when blood begins to flow; fist pumping may increase blood potassium levels and should not be encouraged. Excessively massaging the site or probing or redirecting the needle multiple times may result in hemoconcentration.

83. A: Evacuated tube system (ETS) tubes should always be filled until the normal amount of vacuum is exhausted; partially filling a normal draw sodium fluoride tube or pulling back the plunger on a syringe too quickly may result in hemolysis. Although procedural errors are the most common cause, patient conditions such as liver disease or hemolytic anemia may result in hemolysis.

84. D: Underfilling additive tubes is unacceptable as a time-saving device; underfilling is acceptable when obtaining larger amounts of blood is inadvisable, such as when drawing blood from infants or children or from severely anemic patients. Short draw serum tubes such as red tops and serum separator tubes (SSTs) are acceptable provided the specimen is not hemolyzed and there is enough of the specimen for testing.

85. C: A collapsed vein may result from the vacuum draw of the tube or pressure from pulling on the syringe or if the tourniquet is too tight or too close to the venipuncture site. Stoppage of blood flow when the tourniquet is removed may simply indicate that the needle is not positioned properly; slightly adjusting the needle usually reestablishes blood flow. Improper needle position may result in rolling veins.

86. B: Capillary puncture is the preferred method for infants and young children due to their smaller blood volume and risk of injury or serious adverse events such as anemia or cardiac arrest and is typically used for newborn screening; however, it is not appropriate for dehydrated patients or those with poor circulation. Capillary puncture cannot be used for coagulation studies, blood cultures, or tests requiring large volumes of serum or plasma.

87. D: The middle or ring finger is the recommended site for capillary puncture; the tip of the finger should not be used due to the short distance between the skin surface and bone nor the index finger because of its increased sensitivity and more frequent use. The big toe is no longer recommended as a site for capillary collection.

88. A: The medial or lateral plantar surface of the heel is the preferred site for capillary puncture; the earlobe or arch or other areas of the foot should not be used for puncture. The posterior curvature of the heel should not be used, as the bone may be only 1 mm deep in this area.

89. C: Warming of the injection site does not significantly affect results of routinely tested analytes; warming is preferred for heelstick procedures in infants due to their high red blood cell counts and is required for collection of blood gas or capillary pH specimens. Warming may be required before fingersticks in patients with cold hands.

90. A: During blood collection, the first drop of blood should be wiped away, as it may be contaminated with tissue fluid or may contain alcohol residue that may hemolyze the specimen or prevent blood from forming a well-rounded drop. Using strong repetitive pressure to milk the site may result in hemolysis or tissue fluid contamination; using a scooping motion against the skin surface may cause platelet clumping or hemolysis. Removing the tube from the site may create air spaces in the specimen that interfere with test results.

91. C: When administering a tuberculosis (TB) skin test, avoid areas of the arm with scars, bruises, burns, or excessive hair because they may interfere with test results. Applying pressure to the site may force the antigen out of the site and wiping the site with gauze may cause the antigen to be absorbed. Applying a bandage to the site may result in fluid absorption or irritation and may affect test results.

92. D: Collection timing is most critical for drugs with short half-lives, such as the aminoglycosides; timing is less critical for drugs with longer half-lives such as phenobarbital or digoxin. Timing is not essential for ethanol or blood alcohol testing.

93. B: During blood alcohol (ethanol) [ETOH] testing, regular soap and water may be used to clean the venipuncture site if an alternative disinfectant such as povidone-iodine or aqueous benzalkonium chloride is not available; disinfectants that contain alcohol such as tincture of iodine, isopropyl alcohol, or methanol should not be used, as they may compromise test results.

94. C: Rickets usually occurs in children and is marked by abnormal or "soft" bones caused by a lack of vitamin D in the diet; arthritis is an inflammatory condition of the joints. Osteochondritis is an inflammation of the bone and cartilage, and osteomyelitis is inflammation of the bone or bone marrow caused by bacterial infection.

95. B: Gout is a form of arthritis affecting the joints of the feet caused by increased uric acid levels in the blood; bursitis is an inflammation of the bursa between the muscle attachments and bone. Rickets is a condition in children caused by lack of vitamin D marked by softening and malformation of the bones; a slipped disc is a condition in which the disc between the vertebrae of the spine ruptures or protrudes out of place.

96. C: The urine culture and sensitivity (C & S) test is used to diagnose cystitis; ACTH is used to assess adrenocorticotropic hormone and thyroid-stimulating hormone (TSH) levels. FBS is the fasting blood sugar test.

97. D: Because type O blood lacks antigens, an individual with type O blood can be a donor to individuals with any of the four blood types; thus, type O blood is known as the universal donor.

98. C: Because type AB blood lacks antibodies in its plasma, an individual with this blood type can receive blood from all 4 blood types; thus, type AB blood is known as the universal recipient.

99. D: The Rh factor is also known as the D antigen.

100. A: Anemia is a condition indicated by a deficiency of red blood cells and hemoglobin in the blood; leukemia is a condition characterized by an increase in the number of white blood cells. Thrombocytopenia is marked by a decrease in the number of platelets and polycythemia an excessive number of red blood cells.

101. B: The butterfly infusion set is used for patients with small, fragile veins, such as the elderly, infants or small children, or adults with small antecubital wrists; it is not used in obese patients.

102. C: Only physicians or specially trained emergency room personnel are qualified to perform arterial puncture; the phlebotomist is not trained to perform this procedure. Patients should be checked for allergies and must be in a steady state; thus, a patient who is afraid of needles must be calmed down before the procedure. The risk of hematoma is increased with arterial puncture.

103. A: Intraoperative blood collection is used for procedures in which the estimated amount of blood loss is 20% or more of the patient's blood volume; it is typically used in patients undergoing cardiac, vascular, gynecologic, trauma, or transplant surgery. Intraoperative blood collection is not used for cancer or lower GI tract surgery or for infants or small children due to the risk of anemia or cardiac arrest.

104. D: An implanted port is attached to an indwelling line and should not be covered with a bandage. A heparin lock is a special type of cannula that can be left in the patient's vein for up to 48 hours; however, coagulation studies should not be drawn from a heparin lock. Arteriovenous (AV) shunts are usually created to provide access for dialysis; venipuncture or blood pressure should not be performed on an AV shunt.

105. B: The pH for arterial blood should be maintained at a level of 7.35 to 7.45.

106. C: A patient's blood glucose level is normally elevated after ingestion of a high-carbohydrate meal; however, glucose levels return to normal within 2 hours after ingestion.

107. A: Normal blood glucose levels for a healthy adult should range from 65 to 110 mg/dL.

108. B: Sodium is the most plentiful electrolyte in serum or plasma.

109. A: Both sodium and potassium play a role in maintaining osmotic pressure and acid-base balance; potassium is important in maintaining muscle function and cardiac output. Blood urea nitrogen (BUN) is used to measure renal function.

110. C: Human chorionic gonadotropin (hCG) levels are increased during pregnancy; however, HCG may not be present in sufficient levels the first week or 2 after conception, and thus may yield false-negative results. Contaminants such as detergents, protein, hematuria, and bacteria as well as certain medications may invalidate results. Malignant ovarian tumors and other conditions may increase HCG levels.

111. A: A long-lasting white foam may indicate renal disease; deeply pigmented yellow foam on yellow-brown or -green urine may indicate the presence of bilirubin or biliverdin, which are associated with hepatitis. Normal urine may range in color from yellow to dark amber. Bacteria and epithelial cells are indicative of a pathological condition only when present in large quantities.

112. D: A positive nitrite test in conjunction with a positive leukocyte test is indicative of urinary tract infection (UTI); a urine culture positive for blood or protein is also indicative of UTI. Glucose in the urine may be indicative of diabetes mellitus.

113. C: Trough levels are collected when the serum concentration of the drug is at its lowest level, usually just prior to administration of the next dose; peak levels are collected when the serum concentration is highest, usually 30 to 60 minutes after drug administration, and are used to screen for drug intoxication. Neither peak nor trough levels are useful for DNA testing.

114. B: The purified protein derivative (PPD) skin test is used to diagnose tuberculosis (TB); the Schick test is used in the diagnosis of diphtheria and the Dick test in the diagnosis of scarlet fever. The histoplasmosis (histo) test is used to test for infection with the organism Histoplasmosis capsulatum.

115. C: Prior to a fecal occult blood test, patients are prohibited from ingesting foods such as red meat, turnips, horseradish, vitamin C, aspirin, or anti-inflammatory drugs; however, patient are encouraged to eat fruits such as prunes, grapes, or apples and vegetables such as spinach, lettuce, and corn.

116. B: Bilirubin is normally present in the blood but not in the urine and is indicative of liver or gallbladder disease or cancer. Albumin is the primary protein found in urine; ketones are end products of fat metabolism and normally present in the urine. Bacteria may be present in the urine in small amounts; only large quantities of bacteria are indicative of pathology.

117. D: Cryoglobulin, cryofibrinogen, and cold agglutinin specimens must be kept at or near body temperature; lactic acid, ammonia, and glucagon specimens require chilling.

118. C: The transverse plane divides the body into top and bottom halves; the sagittal plane divides the body into unequal right and left halves and the midsagittal plane into equal right and left halves. The frontal plane is parallel to the long axis of the body and at right angles to the midsagittal plane.

119. D: The abbreviation q stands for "every"; thus, Q2H means that the drug should be given every 2 hours. BID indicates that the drug should be administered twice a day and PO means given orally (from the Latin per os), or by mouth.

120. A: Connective tissue is the most common type of tissue found in the body; muscle tissue is essential for movement and epithelial tissue protects the internal and external structures of the body. Nerve tissue consists of cells that send and receive information.

121. C: There are a total of 206 bones in the human body.

122. B: There are a total of 656 muscles in the body.

123. C: The synapse is the area between neurons over which impulses literally jump to transmit messages; dendrites and axons are extensions of the neuron. The myelin sheath covers the axon and increases the speed of a nerve impulse.

124. B: The white matter of the brain is composed of the myelin sheath; nonmyelinated axons are not covered by the myelin sheath and are known as the gray matter. Schwann cells are a fatty substance that composes the myelin sheath; synapses are areas between neurons over which impulses jump to transmit messages.

125. A: The peripheral nervous system (PNS) is located outside of the central nervous system (CNS) and is composed of the cranial nerves except the optic nerve, the spinal nerves, and the autonomic nervous system. The spinal cord and brain compose the CNS.

126. D: Hydrocephalus is an increased volume of cerebrospinal fluid in the brain at birth and is characterized by an enlargement of the infant's head; headache, stiff neck, and fever are symptoms of meningitis, or an inflammation of the meninges of the brain. A shuffling gait, muscular rigidity, and tremor are characteristic of Parkinson disease, and nerve pain is characteristic of neuralgia.

127. B: The outermost layer of the skin is known as the epidermis; the second layer, or the dermis, is thicker than the epidermis and is known as the "true skin." The subcutaneous or hypodermal layer lies underneath the dermis.

128. C: Hiatal hernia is a condition marked by protrusion of the stomach through a weak area of the diaphragm; gastritis is an acute or chronic inflammation of the stomach lining, and peptic ulcer is erosion of the stomach lining. Gastroesophageal reflux disease (GERD) is a relaxation of the lower sphincter muscle that allows the contents of the stomach to move up the esophagus.

129. D: Sweat glands are a type of exocrine gland, which is composed of ducts that carry secretions to the body surface or to organs. The pancreas, pituitary, and thyroid are endocrine glands, or ductless glands that secrete hormones directly into the bloodstream.

130. B: Dwarfism is caused by hypofunctioning of the pituitary gland in childhood; Cushing syndrome is caused by hypersecretion of the glucocorticoid hormone and diabetes by reduced secretion of insulin from the pancreas. Parkinson disease is a disorder of the peripheral nervous system.

131. C: The throat is also known as the pharynx; the larynx is known as the voice box, and the trachea is known as the windpipe. The epiglottis is a covering of the opening of the larynx that causes food to pass down the esophagus rather than the trachea.

132. A: Asthma is caused by obstruction of the airway due to inflammation; bronchitis is caused by inflammation of the bronchial tubes. Hyperventilation is characterized by rapid breathing resulting in a loss of carbon dioxide. Hypoxia is caused by oxygen deficiency.

133. C: The major portion of the heart is known as the myocardium; the pericardium is a layer of fibrous tissue that surrounds the heart, and the endocardium covers the inner layer of the heart. The atrium is the receiving chamber of the heart.

134. A: The ventricles are the chambers of the heart that pump blood; the right ventricle pumps deoxygenated blood to the lungs and the left oxygenated blood to the rest of the body. The atria are the chambers of the heart that receive blood. The endocardium covers the inner layer of the heart; the septum is the wall of cartilage that separates the four chambers.

135. C: The human body has an average of 8 to 10 pints, or 4 to 5 quarts, of blood.

136. D: Approximately 92% of plasma is composed of water; the remainder is composed of solutes. Fibrinogen is a plasma protein; electrolytes such as sodium, calcium, and potassium come from food and are found in plasma in smaller amounts.

137. C: Aspartate aminotransferase (AST) is typically used to diagnose cardiovascular conditions. Hemoglobin (Hgb), complete blood count (CBC), and erythrocyte sedimentation rate (ESR) are used to diagnose blood diseases such as anemia or leukemia.

138. B: The arterial puncture site is typically used for testing arterial blood gases (ABGs); the antecubital veins are used for venipuncture, with the median cubital vein considered the first choice. The veins located in the antecubital fossa are used for venous puncture.

139. C: A suprapubic specimen may be collected for infants or small children to ensure that the sample is not contaminated; the clean catch and midstream clean catch methods are used for adults to ensure an uncontaminated specimen. For a regular void specimen, urine is simply collected in a wide-mouth container.

140. D: Tests for cerebrospinal fluid (CSF) include total protein, glucose, and chloride; ABO typing is used for paternity testing.

141. B: A postprandial (PP) specimen is collected 2 hours after ingestion of a meal; fasting blood sugar (FBS) testing occurs after the patient has fasted 12 hours. Hgb, or hemoglobin, may be collected regardless of meals. HBV stands for hepatitis B virus.

142. C: The prothrombin time (PT) test may be used in conjunction with partial thromboplastin time (PTT) to assess a patient's total clotting abnormalities; activated coagulation time (ACT) is used to monitor heparin therapy. APPT stands for activated partial thromboplastin time and PP postprandial testing.

143. B: As with prothrombin time (PT), activated partial thromboplastin time (APPT) whole blood values differ from plasma values; normal whole blood values range from 93 to 127 seconds and normal plasma values from 24 to 34 seconds.

144. A: Blood gas values such as partial pressure of carbon dioxide (pCO2) are typically ordered stat; human chorionic gonadotropin (hCG) is a pregnancy test. The fasting blood sugar (FBS) test is a timed test for which patients must restrict dietary intake for 12 hours. The hemoglobin (Hgb) test is used to diagnose anemia.

145. C: Enteric isolation procedures are required for patients with intestinal infections that may be transmitted by ingestion; drainage/secretion isolation is required for burn patients or those with skin infections. AFB (acid-fast-bacilli) isolation is used for patients with tuberculosis.

146. D: The Occupational Safety and Health Administration (OSHA) requires that a high-efficiency particulate air (HEPA) respirator be used to protect healthcare workers caring for acid-fast-bacilli (AFB) patients, such as those with infectious tuberculosis; a HEPA respirator is not required for enteric or contact isolation patients or burn patients.

147. C: The Occupational Safety and Health Administration (OSHA) requires manufacturers of hazardous chemicals to supply Safety Data Sheets (SDS) for all chemical products; SDS are kept in a laboratory logbook or binder as a reference for lab personnel.

148. A: Contaminated needles should never be recapped; the phlebotomist should replace the patient's bed rails after specimen collection and report unusual odors, spills, or dropped items to the nurse.

149. C: Environmental conditions such as water, oxygen or lack of oxygen, proper pH, darkness, and proper temperature of 37.5ºC or 98.6ºF are required for pathogen growth.

150. B: Postexposure treatment with hepatitis B immune globulin (HBIG) is effective in preventing HBV; however, no vaccine is available for either HCV or HIV.

151. C: Because exposure does not necessarily lead to human immunodeficiency virus (HIV), as well as the potential for serious drug side effects, postexposure treatment is not recommended for all occupational exposures to HIV. No vaccine is available for HIV, and HIV may be transmitted through breast milk. Those exposed to HIV should be tested 6 weeks, 12 weeks, and 6 months after exposure.

152. B: The reservoir host is a person, animal, plant, or other organism or substance that acts as the source of transmission of a pathogen; the susceptible host is the person capable of being infected with a pathogen. The chain of infection is the order in which pathogens are transmitted; direct contact is the direct physical transfer of pathogens from a reservoir to a susceptible host.

153. D: Personal protective equipment (PPE) such as gloves, mask, and gowns is required when entering the room of a patient under drainage/secretion isolation, such as those with skin infections, AFB isolation, such as those with tuberculosis, or enteric isolation, such as those with intestinal infections that may be transmitted through ingestion; PPE is not required for patients with HIV.

154. C: Some chemicals may be activated by water and should not be flushed; the safety data sheets (SDS) should be consulted for detailed information regarding antidotes. Mixing bleach and ammonia creates a gas that may be toxic. Electrical hazards should be moved away from the patient using a broom handle or another object made of glass or wood. Lead aprons and lead-lined gloves are required as a precaution against radioactive hazards.

155. B: The accession number, time of test, patient's name and date of birth, and the phlebotomist's initials are required information on specimen tube labels; the physician's signature is required on requisition forms.

156. D: Laboratory requisition forms may be transmitted to the laboratory via courier, pneumatic tube system, or in the case of computerized forms, e-mail; verbal laboratory requests may only be given in the outpatient or emergency setting and must be documented on a laboratory requisition form.

157. B: When taking calls, the phlebotomist should not wait until the first call is finished before taking another call; ask the first caller for permission to be put on hold, then answer the second call. When the second call is completed, return to the first call. An individual's "personal space," or comfort zone, is based on culture and should be respected. Sign language may be used for both hearing-impaired and non–English-speaking patients.

158. C: Negligence is defined as the failure to act, resulting in injury or harm to the patient, and does not require intent to harm. Invasion of privacy is a tort involving use of a patient's name for commercial gain, intrusion into a patient's private life, or disclosure of private information. Abandonment is the premature termination of a professional relationship with a patient without notice or patient consent.

159. A: Abandonment, or the premature termination of a professional relationship between a healthcare provider and a patient without notice or patient consent, is an example of an intentional tort; negligence does not require intent. Malpractice is negligence or improper treatment by a health care professional. Chain of custody refers to the procedure for ensuring that specimens have been obtained for the correct patient, have been labeled correctly, and have not been subject to tampering.

160. C: Pre- and post- are examples of a prefix, which is added to the beginning of a word to indicate an amount, location, or time; pre- means "before" and post- means "after." A suffix is added to the end of a word and indicates a procedure, condition, or disease, such as "-algia," or pain. An abbreviation is used to shorten a medical term, such as "BID," or twice a day. A root word is the basis of a term and establishes its meaning; for example, "cardi" is a root word meaning heart.

161. D: The term caudal means toward the tail, or inferior; cranial means toward the head, or superior. The term medial means toward the midline, and lateral means toward the side of the body.

162. C: Glass tubes are preferred for blood alcohol specimens because of the porous nature of plastic tubes; random drug screening may be performed without patient consent, such as in the case of athletes or employees of health care organizations. A split sample may be required for confirmation or parallel testing. A proctor may be required to be present to verify that the specimen was obtained from the correct individual.

163. B: The activated clotting time (ACT) test is used to monitor heparin levels; partial pressure of oxygen (PO2) is an arterial blood gas and ionized calcium an electrolyte. Glucose levels are measured by the 2-hour postprandial (PP) test.

164. D: Arsenic, zinc, iron, copper, aluminum, and lead are all examples of trace elements; magnesium is not a trace element.

165. B: Measurement of cardiac troponin is useful in the diagnosis of acute myocardial infarction or heart attack; glucose testing is used in diagnosing diabetes. Hematocrit is used for anemia and occult blood for colon cancer screening.

166. C: B-type natriuretic peptide (BNP) blood concentrations are measured to detect congestive heart failure; the purified protein derivative (PPD) skin test is used to test for tuberculosis. The Histo and Cocci skin tests are used to test for the fungal infections Histoplasmosis and Coccidioidomycosis, respectively.

167. B: In administering a tuberculosis (TB) skin test, the antigen should be injected just below the skin, not into a vein. Presence of a bleb or wheal indicates that the antigen was injected properly. A TB reaction is measured according to the degree of induration or hardness, not erythema or redness.

168. C: A positive reaction to a TB skin test is indicated by induration of 10 mm or greater in diameter; induration between 5 and 9 mm in diameter indicates a doubtful reaction and less than 5 mm in diameter a negative reaction. The degree of redness or erythema is not relevant.

169. D: The first step in performing a test for group A streptococci is nitrous acid or enzymatic extraction of the throat swab specimen, followed by latex agglutination or enzyme immunoassay for antigen detection. Specific gravity is measured through urinalysis.